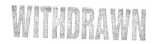

Infectious Behavior

Infectious Behavior

Brain-Immune Connections in Autism, Schizophrenia, and Depression

Paul H. Patterson

The MIT Press
Cambridge, Massachusetts
London, England

© 2011 Massachusetts Institute of Technology

All rights reserved. No part of this book may be reproduced in any form by any electronic or mechanical means (including photocopying, recording, or information storage and retrieval) without permission in writing from the publisher.

For information about special quantity discounts, please e-mail special_sales@ mitpress.mit.edu

This book was set in Stone Sans and Stone Serif by Toppan Best-set Premedia Limited. Printed and bound in the United States of America.

Library of Congress Cataloging-in-Publication Data

Patterson, Paul H.
Infectious behavior : brain-immune connections in autism, schizophrenia, and depression / Paul H. Patterson.
  p. ; cm.
Includes bibliographical references and index.
ISBN 978-0-262-01645-2 (hardcover : alk. paper)
1. Mental illness—Immunological aspects. 2. Psychology, Pathological. I. Title.
[DNLM: 1. Mental Disorders—immunology. 2. Brain—embryology.
3. Brain—immunology. 4. Immune System—physiopathology. 5. Maternal-Fetal Exchange. WM 100]
RC454.4.P38 2011
616.89′071—dc22

2011006509

10 9 8 7 6 5 4 3 2 1

To Carolyn and Paul Clair for their inspiration and patience

Contents

Acknowledgments   ix

Introduction   xi

1 Fever and Madness   1

2 Brain-Immune Connections, Stress, and Depression   9

3 The Battleground of the Fetal-Maternal Environment   29

4 Prenatal Origins of Adult Health and Disease   43

5 Infections and Behavior   61

6 Animal Models of Autism, Schizophrenia, and Depression?   73

7 Immune Involvement in Autism, Schizophrenia, and Depression   99

8 Pre- and Postnatal Vaccination: Risks and Benefits   117

9 Reasons for Optimism   129

Perspectives   149

Further Reading   151

Index   157

Acknowledgments

I am delighted to have the opportunity to thank my wife, Carolyn, for her careful and thoughtful editorial comments on this material. Elaine Hsiao produced the informative and attractive original illustrations, and Laura Rodriguez provided excellent editorial assistance. Ali Khoshnan, Suzanne York, and River Malcolm made useful comments on early versions of several chapters. Alan Brown, Carlos Pardo, and David Barker made time for extended conversations about their areas of considerable expertise. Alan has also provided numerous mini-tutorials in epidemiology over the years, and we collaborated recently on the new book *The Origins of Schizophrenia*, published by Columbia University Press. I also wish to thank the members of my laboratory at Caltech, who have produced much useful data over the years on neuroimmune interactions and on the maternal infection risk factor. Several faculty colleagues and collaborators, past and present, have also contributed materially and intellectually to the story presented here.

Introduction

This book is intended for those in the general public who are interested in new advances in our understanding of how the brain works, as well as those who have a particular interest in autism, schizophrenia, or depression. One novel aspect of the book is its focus on the bidirectional cross talk between the brain and the immune system. These neuroimmune interactions are described as they occur in healthy people as well as in those with mental disorders. Another theme that runs through the book involves the interactions between the mother and her fetus. This is an important topic because maternal-fetal interactions are essential for the development of normal behavior in the offspring, and they are critical in the development of the behaviors and neuropathology that we call mental illness. The roles of immune cells and immune-related molecules are illuminated by way of information gleaned from a wide variety of animal and human studies.

I arrived at this book from several directions. First, my laboratory's research accidentally veered into the interactions between the nervous and immune systems. For many years, we had worked on characterizing a protein that had the amazing ability to change the fate of developing neurons. That is, when the protein was added to those neurons, in cultures with cardiac muscle cells, the neurons went from being excitatory (speeding up the heartbeat) to inhibitory (slowing it down). When we obtained the sequence of the gene that codes for this interesting protein, we found its sequence to be identical to one recently obtained for a protein that had important effects on cells of the immune system. That the same protein could operate in both the nervous and immune systems suggested that it could mediate cross talk between the two systems. In fact, subsequent work has shown that this protein is indeed important in mediating inflammatory reactions within the brain. This line of investigation led our laboratory into the field of what came to be known as neuroimmune interaction. It also helped lead to the identification of an entire family of similar proteins that can mediate neuroimmune functions.

The second impetus for this book arose from lectures on mental illness that I gave while on the faculty at Harvard Medical School and later at the California Institute of Technology. I became particularly interested in schizophrenia, a complex but fascinating disorder, and was disappointed in the animal models that were available at the time. Knowing how effective the use of truly appropriate animal models can be in studies of disease, our laboratory set out to see if we could make a contribution in this area. Because work with animal models of mental illness was seen by some as "soft science," and known as an extremely difficult area in which to make rapid progress, some of my colleagues attempted to discourage me from starting such a project. Nonetheless, I shared the opinion of a former president of the Society for Neuroscience, Huda Akil of the University of Michigan, that "studying the neurobiology of mental illness is not a luxury that neuroscientists can engage in after they have handled more accessible problems." And I firmly believe, as do the writers of a recent editorial in the journal *Nature*, that "there are many ways in which the understanding and treatment of conditions such as schizophrenia are ripe for a revolution." In fact, such a revolution is currently under way. This is readily apparent from some of the new findings summarized in this book.

The key point of entry for me was reading about the epidemiology work investigating possible causes of schizophrenia. The fact that many studies pointed to infections in pregnant women as a risk factor for schizophrenia in the offspring suggested a straightforward experiment in mice: could maternal infection lead to offspring with features of mental illness? The parallel question was, of course, could features of mental illness be observed in mice? We proceeded to show that the behaviors of the offspring of infected pregnant mice were consistent with some of the behaviors seen in schizophrenia, and this launched our laboratory into the study of how maternal infection influences fetal brain development. In this roundabout way, a second part of our group came to be working on neuroimmune interactions.

A third motive for this book came from the work of many investigators who are uncovering evidence of immune involvement in schizophrenia, major depressive disorder, and autism. I believe that such work is not yet fully appreciated by the biomedical community, overshadowed as it is, in both publicity and funding, by genetic approaches to these diseases. Moreover, my experience in giving lectures for the general public has shown me that even laypersons with an active interest in biomedical science are generally unaware of the important connections between the mind and the immune system, and of the role in mental illness played by the immune-related molecules and cells described here. The book is intended for those readers.

My enthusiasm for this research, and for the book, was further propelled by an autism diagnosis in our nephew and by the compelling work of my wife, Carolyn Patterson, who very effectively teaches children with special needs, including many with autism.

In this short book I have chosen to combine these various threads in the following manner. Chapter 1, "Fever and Madness," brings a historical perspective to immune manipulations in the treatment of mental illness, highlighting the frightening but fascinating experiments from the early days of the study of the mind-body connection. Chapter 2, "Brain-Immune Connections, Stress, and Depression," describes how the immune system influences behavior and how the brain regulates the immune system. The ways in which this bidirectional cross talk influences stress and major depressive disorder are considered, and some of the molecules involved are introduced. Emphasis is given to findings that neuroimmune interactions operate both when people and animals are healthy and during periods of disease or injury.

Because many aspects of mental illness have their origins in early fetal brain development, we also delve into relevant aspects of embryology. Chapter 3, "The Battleground of the Fetal-Maternal Environment," considers the role of immune cells and inflammatory molecules in fetal development, and the immunological paradox of pregnancy: why is the fetus not seen as foreign, and rejected by the maternal immune system? The possible role of hormones in the development of autism in utero is also considered. Chapter 4, "Prenatal Origins of Adult Health and Disease," explains the concept of fetal programming and how it can lead to adult disease. Newly discovered molecular mechanisms whereby mental traits can be passed down through generations are described. The next chapter, "Infections and Behavior," examines a different influence on fetal brain outcome—maternal infection. How can infection in the pregnant woman influence mood, behavior, and disease in the offspring? A variety of maternal infections are discussed in the context of both schizophrenia and autism. The difficult question of how experiments on animals can tell us anything about disorders such as autism and schizophrenia is taken up in chapter 6, "Animal Models of Autism, Schizophrenia, and Depression?" Can the symptoms of these disorders really be assessed in rodents? We consider models of genetic and environmental risk factors for these disorders, along with the role of inflammation and immune-related molecules.

The considerable body of evidence that the immune system is involved in mental disorders is the central topic of chapter 7, "Immune Involvement in Autism, Schizophrenia, and Depression." The roles of antibodies, cytokines, and even the gastrointestinal tract are considered. Since immune activation is highly relevant for these disorders, the next chapter, "Pre- and Postnatal Vaccination: Risks and Benefits," takes on the hot topic of the risks and benefits of both pre- and postnatal vaccinations. Since much of the book considers the numerous ways in which things can go wrong and lead to mental illness, it is appropriate to end with chapter 9, "Reasons for Optimism," which describes recent experiments indicating that both early postnatal and adult interventions can lead to positive outcomes. In particular, evidence from animal models is leading to a number of promising clinical trials for treatment of neurodevelopmental disorders.

For questions for the author and updates on the various topics covered in the book since its publication, please check the book's website: http://mitpress.mit.edu/infectiousbehavior.

1 Fever and Madness

Although the "Spanish flu" pandemic lasted for only a year, its dark legacy still haunts us. The year 1918 saw the appearance of the novel strain of influenza virus called H1N1, which caused the most widespread and lethal flu infection in recorded history (figure 1.1). An estimated 20 to 100 million people died worldwide. It killed more Americans in one year than died in all the wars of the twentieth century. Surprisingly, this virus was especially lethal for the healthiest in the population—young adults, and particularly, pregnant women. Interestingly, this was also true of the recent pandemic virus of 2009. Because of the work of Jeffrey Taubenberger and colleagues at the Armed Forces Institute of Pathology in Washington, D.C., we now know quite a bit about the 1918 virus. Taubenberger and Ann Reid used tissue that had been preserved in formaldehyde and paraffin from soldiers who died of the flu in 1918, and Johan Hultin retrieved tissue from Eskimos who died of the flu that year and were buried in the permafrost, which preserved the virus. Sequencing the genes of this lethal virus has revealed that it probably was derived from an influenza virus that infected birds, and through mutation, became able to infect mammals such as pigs and people. This remarkable virus still casts its ominous shadow today: its descendants have continued to cause pandemics or global outbreaks such as those in 1947, 1951, 1957, 1968, 1997, and 2003. The global pandemic in 2009 was caused by a fourth-generation descendant of the bird-swine-human influenza virus of 1918.

Far less appreciated, however, is another sinister, decades-long legacy left by this virus. A graduate student at Columbia University and the National Bureau of Economic Research, Douglas Almond, used a remarkably simple method of uncovering the continuing human costs of the 1918 pandemic. In addition to the obvious effects on families from the loss of

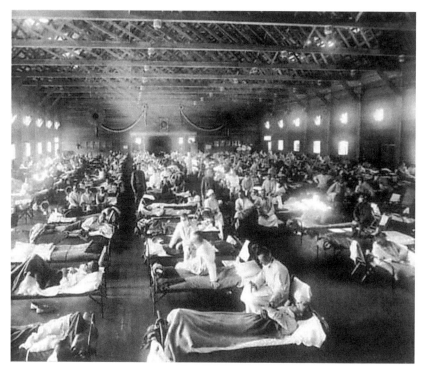

Figure 1.1
The huge numbers of patients struck down by the 1918 pandemic had to be warehoused in large dormitories, often lacking adequate care. (Photo courtesy of the National Museum of Health and Medicine, Armed Forces Institute of Pathology, Washington, D.C.)

mothers or fathers, there were hidden effects on the fetuses gestating at the time the pandemic swept through the United States. Some of those effects did not become clear until the fetuses became adults. Using the socioeconomic data collected each decade by the U.S. Census Bureau, Almond discovered that the offspring of women who were pregnant precisely during the time the flu came through their area grew up to have lower income, socioeconomic status, and educational attainment than those who had been gestating just before or after the pandemic. These effects suggest that the virus affected fetal brain development. Other data indicate that this group also had higher rates of physical disability, heart disease, and diabetes. Thus, more than sixty years later, this group of offspring was still suffering the consequences of the pandemic. These results support the more general "fetal origins of adult disease" hypothesis, which arises from studies showing that a number of disorders, such as cardio-vascular disease and diabetes, are associated with problems experienced by the mother during fetal development. This hypothesis is the subject of chapter 4.

As we shall see in chapter 5, infection of pregnant women also increases the risk of mental illness in the offspring. Research on this association is particularly strong for schizophrenia, where the initial hospitalization for psychosis typically occurs in late adolescence or early adulthood. Thus, it is another example of the fetal origins of adult disease syndrome. In this case, the outcome is related to the mother's inflammatory response to various types of infection, including influenza. In fact, the connection between infection, immune reactions, and psychosis has been investigated and hotly debated for more than a hundred years. The most striking experimental studies done on humans in this context were carried out at the turn of the last century by Julius Wagner-Jauregg (see figure 1.2), who received the Nobel Prize in 1927 for his work on "pyrotherapy" (fever therapy). He had noted as early as 1883 during his psychiatry residency in the Vienna Asylum that some patients experiencing psychiatric symp-toms such as hallucinations, mania, depression, paranoia, apathy, and severe disorientation displayed a marked improvement while they were sick with infections such as those caused by streptococcus, tuberculosis, or typhoid. The relationship between fever and "madness" had been dis-cussed over the centuries, but Wagner-Jauregg made the critical step toward clinical experimentation when he began to treat patients by manipulating their immune systems (figure 1.3). Interestingly, his first approach was to give patients tuberculin, which was tested as a treatment for tuberculosis by the famous German microbiologist Robert Koch in 1890. While tuber-culin turned out to be ineffective for treating tuberculosis, this extract of tubercle bacteria is still used today in a skin test to detect tuberculosis infec-tion. That is, if one has been infected by the tubercle bacterium, injection of tuberculin generates a strong inflammatory response caused by the immune system's memory of seeing this protein previously during the infection. Wagner-Jauregg reported that tuberculin injection caused long-term remission of psychotic and other symptoms of syphilis, which were called the "general paresis of the insane," or dementia paralytica. Thinking that this worked by causing fever, Wagner-Jauregg switched to giving such

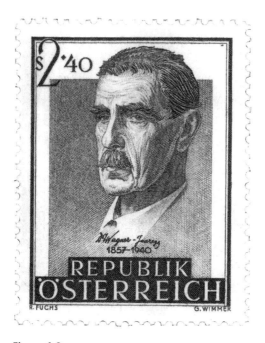

Figure 1.2
Austria issued this commemorative stamp for the one-hundredth anniversary of
Wagner-Jauregg's birth in 1857. Although many schools and streets had been named
for him, the later discovery that Wagner-Jauregg was a proponent of racial purity
and Nazi ideology evoked a reexamination of his heroic status in modern Austria.
(Reproduced with permission from *J Neurol Neurosurg Psychiat* 62:3, 1997)

patients malaria infections, which may have elicited stronger and more
reproducible fevers.

In June 1917, the initial experiment involved taking blood from a
soldier with malaria and injecting it into a 37-year-old actor with advanced
symptoms of syphilis. After three weeks, the patient had his first fever
episode, followed by nine more such malaria attacks. Incredibly, after the
sixth fever episode, the "syphilis fits" ended, and the patient recovered
completely from both malaria and syphilis. He was discharged from the
asylum that December. Wagner-Jauregg applied the same regime to nine
more patients. Three of these were discharged as being cured of dementia
paralytica, three improved but later worsened, two experienced no change
in psychosis, one developed a severe "paralytic melancholy," and another
died of malaria. Wagner-Jauregg concluded that six of the nine had

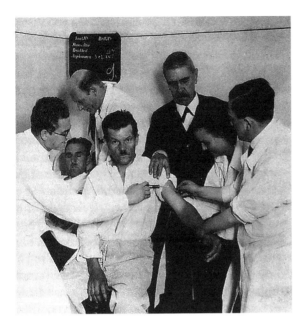

Figure 1.3
Julius Wagner-Jauregg (dark suit) supervises the injection of blood taken from a patient with malaria (rear, lying down) into a psychiatric patient (center). This "pyrotherapy" is thought to have been the first successful physical therapy in psychiatry. (Reproduced with permission from the Department und Sammlungen fur Geschichte der Medizin, Medizinische Universitat Wien)

improved far more than if they had been left untreated, and he published his results the following year. The experiment was a major event in the history of psychiatry, demonstrating that organic or physical treatments could be of value for previously hopeless cases of "madness." While this type of treatment clearly violated the present-day first rule of medicine, to "do no harm," one can argue that it "broke the therapeutic nihilism that had dominated psychiatry in previous generations" (Shorter, 1997). That is, it helped establish the mind-body connection and affirm the possibility of gaining relief through physical treatments.

Given its apparent success in treating dementia paralytica, a few clinicians went on to test the malaria pyrotherapy on schizophrenia patients. In Bristol, England, in the early 1920s, W. L. Templeton tried the by then standard malarial infection strategy on 20 chronic, institutionalized patients and described a truly amazing transformation:

The most striking change was seen in a brightening of intellectual interest, a desire to converse, to read the newspapers and books, and in some, a complete return to normal as far as could be judged. Many began to write letters home, and these revealed a wonderful transformation of interest. Some who had previously refused to interview their relatives welcomed them and discussed past events in a more or less rational way.

However, after two months, when the fever had disappeared, "there were few who had not materially lapsed." The conclusion was eloquent but depressing: "It must be confessed that the earlier results have but flattered to deceive, and it seems as if little or no permanent improvement can be expected from this line of treatment." A similar conclusion was reached by Leland Hinsie, working at the New York State Psychiatric Institute on Ward's Island. Although malaria treatment of 13 schizophrenic patients resulted in several of the patients exhibiting signs of improvement, such as a renewed interest in relatives and engaging in rational conversation with visitors for the first time in years, the change was transient. Hinsie concluded, "We are not encouraged to recommend the malarial form of treatment under the conditions that we have outlined. On the contrary, we feel that there are definite contraindications, these being, first the [increased] mortality rate, and, second, the tendency to arousing latent tuberculous processes which are known to be prevalent in this class of [institutionalized] patients."

Either because of the inherently dangerous nature of the malaria treatment, or the discouraging long-term outcome found in these and a few other small studies, this line of investigation died out over the next few decades. The approach was abandoned despite the fact that the malaria treatment was successfully extended to thousands of syphilis patients during this time and was tested in many other incurable diseases. It is surprising that nothing further was made of the seemingly remarkable, even if transient, improvement seen in some of the fever-treated schizophrenia patients. Although the Templeton and Hinsie experiments, plus a few others, were very small clinical trials, and no control groups were treated with other types of proteins or blood (to test whether the positive effects were due to the blood having come specifically from an infected person), these investigators may have stumbled upon something important. Could it be that the immune system is involved in *maintaining* the psychotic symptoms? Could perturbing this system in this terribly crude way, by using infection, tip the balance back to normality, restoring mental status in a temporary fashion? These topics are taken up in chapters 5 and 7.

The papers of that era suggest that the investigators were focused on the microbes that caused infection rather than on the immune system's responses to those microbes. The latter was the line of investigation taken up by Henry A. Cotton, who worked at the New Jersey State Hospital at Trenton, originally named the New Jersey State Lunatic Asylum. In pursuit of this "focal infection theory" in the early 1920s, Cotton started a controversial program of radical surgical procedures in an attempt to rid psychotic patients of infections that were the putative source of toxins affecting the brain. His surgeries started with the extraction of teeth, but then extended to removal of tissues such as the cervix, ovaries, seminal vesicles, and colon, among others. In 1923, negative results from a carefully controlled study using Cotton's methods finally put this barbaric approach to rest.

However, perhaps thinking along similar lines, Robert Carroll, in 1935 the medical director of the Highland Hospital in Ashville, North Carolina, injected "inactivated" (heated) horse serum into the cerebral spinal fluid of schizophrenics. This was said to be an attempt to test a theory that these patients suffered from low levels of white blood cells. Although positive results were reported, these extremely crude attempts to manipulate the immune system did not lead to further lines of productive investigation during that period.

As we shall see, some of today's more adventurous clinical investigators are picking up these forgotten threads, providing intriguing results on the effects of fever on autism, and even proposing vaccination for schizophrenia and severe depression (chapter 7).

2 Brain-Immune Connections, Stress, and Depression

Over the years your bodies become like walking autobiographies, telling friends and strangers alike of the minor and major stresses of your lives.
—M. Ferguson

If depression is creeping up and must be faced, learn something about the beast: You may escape without a mauling.
—R. W. Shepard

"Happy people make for healthy people," says the wellness Web site. Can positive thinking actually help the immune system to reject tumor cells, or is this merely New Age marketing? Are there genuine, functional connections between the brain and the immune system? If so, what do they do?

Proteins Discovered in the Immune System Can Have Similar Functions in the Brain

A variety of interesting proteins are shared between the immune and nervous systems. A recent discovery of this phenomenon involves the *major histocompatibility complex*, or MHC. These proteins were originally named for their ability to regulate the acceptance of transplanted tissue (*histos*, tissue). That is, tissue can be recognized as foreign or as belonging to oneself, by immune cells that decipher and interpret the MHC proteins found on the cell surfaces of the newly introduced tissue. (The immune system becomes "educated" as to what is "self" at a very young age.) The classical MHC proteins function in cell-mediated immunity: viral or bacterial coat proteins are broken down inside the cell and MHC proteins bind the resulting peptides derived from the invading microbes. The MHC proteins take these peptides to the cell surface, where they "present" or show them to *cytotoxic lymphocytes*. If the peptide is seen as foreign, the cytotoxic lymphocyte can kill the presenting cell (hence the name, cytotoxic). Thus, if a cell is infected with a virus, and its MHC protein presents a peptide from that virus on the cell surface, the presenting cell will be killed, which effectively stops that cell from being a host for viral replication.

Mistakes in this process can result in autoimmune disease, wherein inflammatory cells mistake self for foreign. This can occur if the structure of the viral peptide is the same as a peptide in the human body. In that case, the cytotoxic lymphocytes may kill cells producing the virus, but may also kill other cells in the body with that same peptide on their surface. This phenomenon is termed *molecular mimicry*. Some researchers feel that this is what happens in the autoimmune disease multiple sclerosis. Perhaps the patient was infected with a virus that shared a peptide with the cells that *myelinate*, or insulate nerves. This insulation is critical for the ability of the nerves to conduct or propagate electrical impulses. If cytotoxic lymphocytes mistake the myelinating cells of a nerve for cells that are producing viruses, they may attack and kill those cells. This can result in the loss of electrical conduction in that nerve, which leads to loss of vision or paralysis of limbs. Examples of other autoimmune diseases include diabetes type 1, Crohn's disease (a type of inflammatory bowel disease), Guillain-Barré syndrome (a type of paralysis usually caused by infection), and rheumatoid arthritis. If molecular mimicry is indeed involved in these disorders, it would be another example of the dark legacy of an earlier microbial infection. Such a mechanism has not yet been definitively proven, however.

Some of the current treatments for autoimmune disease involve suppressing the immune response, as can be done with corticosteroid hormones. This type of nonspecific suppression is also used in treating allergies and asthma. A more specific treatment is to block the particular *cytokines* (from the Greek: *cyto*, cell; and *kinos*, movement) that are mediating the attack on the body's cells. Cytokines are small proteins that communicate between cells in the immune system. As we shall see, these proteins are also used in the brain. Cytokine functions can be blocked by administration of antibodies directed against them; the antibodies bind the cytokine, preventing it from recognizing its natural receptor. Alternatively, antibodies that block a cytokine receptor itself, such as the receptor for interleukin-6 (IL-6), are used. Such approaches are being used to treat multiple sclerosis and arthritis, for instance. Schizophrenia, it should be noted, is associated with many different autoimmune diseases. That is, a person who has a history of autoimmune disease is more likely to be at risk for schizophrenia. A similar association with autoimmunity or allergies has been found for autism, particularly if the mother has the autoimmune disorder. Viral and other infections in the mother during pregnancy are also associated with schizophrenia and autism, as we shall discuss in chapter 4.

What about MHC proteins in the brain? In a remarkable series of experiments carried out first at the University of California at Berkeley, the group led by Carla Shatz showed that MHC class I proteins are also produced by neurons (see box 2.1). Moreover, the brain contains neurons that produce

Box 2.1
Carla Shatz

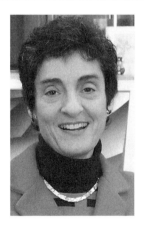

Carla Shatz discovered the presence of the MHC class I system in the brain. She has also made important contributions to our understanding of the early embryonic development of the brain and the visual system. Shatz has shattered a number of glass ceilings in her career, being the first woman to receive a doctorate in neurobiology from Harvard; she later became one of the first female junior faculty and the first tenured woman professor in basic sciences at the Stanford School of Medicine. In 2000 she became the first woman to chair Harvard's neurobiology department—and only the second woman in the history of Harvard Medical School to chair a basic science department. Shatz has returned to Stanford and is currently heading its Bio-X program for interdisciplinary research in biology and medicine. (Photo courtesy of C. J. Shatz)

receptors that bind their MHC partners. Thus, as in the immune system, the MHC system could be used for communication between cells in the brain. It is not clear, however, whether peptide loading of MHC and recognition is involved, as it is, for example, in the immune system for the recognition of pieces of viral proteins (peptides). What Shatz and others have shown so far is that MHC proteins are involved in *synaptic plasticity* during embryonic development. The connections between neurons—the *synapses*—are plastic, or malleable, and can be modified by experience. This is what happens during learning. In fact, mice that lack certain MHC proteins display altered learning capacity. This is shown by experiments in which a gene that codes for an MHC protein is "knocked out," or inactivated. The novel, "knockout" strain of genetically engineered mice is then tested for learning and memory ability. Interestingly, cytokines regulate MHC production in the brain (and in immune cells); this could be one of the ways in which cytokines regulate learning and memory.

An intriguing related finding involving schizophrenia was made by three different groups of geneticists. For many years, and at great expense, large teams of researchers have been searching for genes that predispose people to becoming schizophrenic. A number of such "candidate genes" have been found, although not all studies agree on which ones are most important. Several recent publications identified inherited changes on a site on chromosome 6 as being associated with elevated risk for schizophrenia and bipolar disorder. This chromosomal site is where the MHC genes are located; therefore, the authors suggest that if MHC genes are, in fact, important in schizophrenia, it could be in the context of the immune system, where MHC genes are known to act. In fact, a well-known risk factor for schizophrenia is infection in pregnant women, which increases the chances that the offspring will develop schizophrenia. Some studies have also implicated MHC genes in autism, and there is evidence for a maternal infection link in that disorder as well. The maternal infection risk factor is discussed in chapter 4.

MHC proteins are also important in the formation of connections between the eye and the brain. Before the eyes open, neurons in the retinas of the eyes send long thin processes or extensions, called *axons*, into the brain. Axons from both eyes initially make connections on both sides of the brain. However, when the eyes open and visual function is established, pruning of axons begins, and the synaptic connections made by a great many of the axons are eliminated. The end result is that each eye makes connections predominantly with just one side of the brain. This pruning or elimination of connections is a normal part of development that happens all over the brain, not just in the visual system. The pruning of connections is largely based on which synapses are most active. Those that are less active are lost, while those that are most active are strengthened and enlarged. In the absence of appropriate MHC function, this refinement of connections in the visual system does not occur properly, and the result is miswiring of the pattern of synapses in the visual system.

Another set of immune-related proteins is also involved in the pruning of connections in the visual system. Ben Barres and colleagues at Stanford University found that proteins of the *complement cascade* are necessary for pruning of synapses. When the genes for certain complement proteins are knocked out in mice, there is a failure to properly eliminate synapses during their development. The complement proteins were originally described in the immune system, where they work with antibodies to destroy pathogens. To kill invading bacteria, the complement cascade can actually produce a cylinder that punctures a hole in the bacterial cell membrane. These proteins also stimulate inflammation around the site of the bacterial invasion. In the brain, the complement system is adapted to eliminate inactive synapses, although it is not yet understood how these synapses are marked for destruction. Thus, the complement system has a function in brain development that is analogous to its function in the immune system.

Following the end of the period of synapse elimination, the production of complement proteins declines, so that the normal adult brain contains very low levels of them. However, these levels rise dramatically in the presence of neurodegenerative disease. Complement proteins may be a hundred times the normal level in Alzheimer's disease, for instance. This could be the result of the inflammation that is found in such diseases, and the complement proteins could be contributing to it. These proteins could also be carrying out toxic functions under such circumstances, perhaps eliminating useful synapses or even killing cells. Faulty pruning of synapses also occurs in the developmental disorder known as fragile X syndrome, in which many patients exhibit features of autism. (Fragile X syndrome is described in more detail in chapter 9.)

Other proteins are shared between the immune and nervous systems, and it is intriguing that these various proteins can have analogous functions in the two systems. As mentioned above, the complement system of proteins is used by the immune system to kill invading pathogens, and by the brain to kill synapses. During the evolution of these two systems, functions have been conserved as the same proteins have been adapted for use by immune and neural cells. One consequence of this dual function is that these proteins can allow cross talk between the two systems. Keep in mind, however, that such cross talk can also lead to problems if one of the two systems is diseased—the pathology may spread in this way. One line of defense in preventing this spread is the *blood-brain barrier*, which consists of a series of cells tightly joined together that selectively blocks the access of cells from the blood into the brain. This blood-brain barrier even prevents most large proteins from crossing into the brain. Nonetheless, immune-brain communication is ongoing under normal conditions, as the next section describes.

Immune-to-Brain Communication

Perhaps the most readily apparent example of an immune-brain connection involves the effects of a respiratory virus or an influenza infection on our mental state. If the cold or flu episode is serious enough, typically our behavior changes dramatically—we retreat to bed with a fever, eat little, have disrupted sleep patterns, and socialize hardly at all. Researchers such as Robert Dantzer, formerly of Bordeaux and now at the University of Illinois, have worked out several pathways by which infections can cause such "sickness behavior." Infection by viruses or bacteria activate the immune system, causing inflammatory cells such as lymphocytes to mobilize and kill the invading microbes, and later to make antibodies against the microbes. This mobilization involves signaling between the immune cells, which is done in part by the secretion of cytokines. During infection, the levels of various cytokines such as interleukin-1 (IL-1) and IL-6 rise dramatically near the site of microbe proliferation as well as in the blood and other body fluids. Surprisingly, one of the effects of these cytokines is to activate the vagus nerve, which runs from the brain stem out to a number of internal organs such as the intestines and heart (see figure 2.1). The sickness-driven activation of the vagus by cytokines results in the generation of electrical impulses, which move up the nerve and back into the brain, where, in turn, various other nerve cells (neurons) are activated.

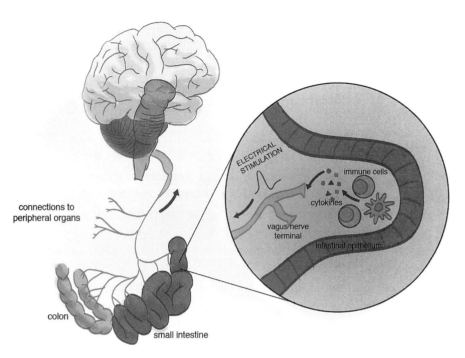

Figure 2.1 (plate 1)
Cytokines evoked by infection, in this case in the gut, stimulate the vagus nerve (yellow) to send electrical signals to the brain. (Illustration by Elaine Hsiao)

At this point something amazing happens: the electrical activity induced by the vagus nerve in specific brain centers is reinterpreted back into a chemical signal—the stimulation of some neurons causes the brain's own immune-like cells, the *microglia*, to produce cytokines—inside the brain! These cytokines bind to their partner receptors on other neurons, as well as to cells in the blood vessels in the brain. This process eventually leads to the changes in behavior that we term "sickness behavior."

We know cytokines are critical in this outcome because of work in animal models. For instance, a rat or mouse can be given an infection, or the infection can be mimicked by injection of molecules made by microbes (the process is similar to a vaccination). These molecules may be components of bacterial cells or viruses; in that scenario no actual living microbe is used. When immune cells detect such molecules, they are activated and produce cytokines. When the experimenter blocks these cytokines in peripheral tissues such as the blood with specific chemical agents, the result is that sickness behavior does not occur. Thus, cytokines produced near the site of infection are required for the eventual sickness behavior produced and governed by the brain. An equally important experiment investigated the role of cytokines within the brain itself. When cytokine inhibitors are injected into the brain, sickness behavior is also blocked. Thus, to induce these behaviors, cytokines are required both in the peripheral tissues out in the far reaches of the body, and within the brain itself. Another lesson here is that peripheral immune activation (by infection in this case) leads to immune activation of the brain, as shown by activation of the brain's microglia and the production of cytokines. Even a single episode of peripheral infection can lead to changes in synaptic connections between neurons in the brain that last for several weeks, and this is likely related to the fact that microglial changes in the brain also last for several weeks.

Activation of the peripheral immune system can also occur in response to other stimuli, such as food allergens or even obesity, which are also associated with immune activation in the brain, as we shall see in later chapters.

These experiments teach us several key lessons. First, immune cells outside the brain can produce signals that alter the activity of neurons within the brain, which results in a specific set of behaviors produced by the animal or human. This insight has led to the investigation of some of the anatomical and chemical pathways that mediate immune-to-brain communication. Second, proteins used for information transfer between immune cells (in this case, cytokines) are also used within the brain for information transfer between neurons. In fact, we also know that cytokines play important signaling roles within the normal brain under healthy conditions. For instance, they are used in the communication between neurons during the formation of memories in the brain. Interestingly, cytokines are also used for communication between immune cells to form *immunological memories*—enabling lymphocytes to respond today to antigens that were encountered by the immune system in the distant past.

A third lesson from these experiments is that animal models can provide essential information for understanding not only how the immune system works and how the brain works, but also how the two systems work together in modifying behavior in adaptive, beneficial ways. "Adaptive" here refers to the supposition that when animals are curled up sick in a burrow (or in bed, in our case), they are less likely to be found in their weakened state by a predator. Their physical inactivity also allows for concentration of metabolic resources in the fight against the infection. So when a person says, "I don't feel good; I'm going to bed," this is the result of a specific sequence of chemical and electrical events that was programmed by evolution in order to protect us during infection. It is also clear that fever itself is adaptive and useful for fighting infection, at least within a normal range. In animal experiments, preventing the induction of fever can result in worsening of infection. A particularly telling experiment showed that cold-blooded animals, which cannot regulate their own body temperature, seek hot conditions such as under a heat lamp when infected. If a lizard, for instance, is not given a heat lamp, its infection will worsen.

Sickness Behavior and Depression

Major depressive disorder has a lifetime prevalence of 20% in women (20% of women will experience the disorder during their lifetime) and 12% in men. Therefore, depression is truly a major public health problem. The disorder is defined by depressed mood lasting more than two weeks, plus disturbed sleep and appetite, feelings of guilt, and suicidal thoughts. Some of these symptoms are, in fact, similar to those found in sickness behavior: lethargy, lack of sociability, cognitive dysfunction, and disordered sleep. This raises the possibility that some of the molecules and neural pathways underlying sickness behavior may be shared with depression. In fact, electrical stimulation of the vagus nerve is now being tested at a few medical centers as a treatment for drug-resistant depression (and for autism). It is not clear how or if this form of stimulation resembles the stimulation of the vagus nerve during infection and sickness behavior, but it is an interesting connection. Another connection is that a key regulator of stress, the peptide known as *corticotropin-releasing factor* (CRF), is elevated in the cerebral spinal fluid in both sickness and depression.

Another striking parallel is illustrated by evidence that cytokines and other molecules associated with inflammation are also involved in depression. For instance, blood levels of pro-inflammatory cytokines such as IL-6 are frequently increased in patients with major depression. It is clear that the increases in cytokines are not merely a side effect of life events. Rather, they can directly affect mood. As discussed in chapter 7 in more detail, injecting patients with cytokines can result in major depressive disorder. Moreover, this cytokine treatment activates the same brain centers that are involved in depression. In the converse approach, clinical trials of cytokine blocking agents have shown that administration of these agents ameliorates depressive symptoms. Major depressive disorder also involves increases in the levels of other markers of immune activation in the blood; moreover, the levels of various types of lymphocytes are altered in the blood of such patients. Several studies have associated inflammation and elevated cytokines in major depression with increased risk of suicide in those subjects. This suggests that appropriate experimental manipulation of immune status could have an effect on this tragic outcome of major depression. In fact, there is evidence that taking aspirin or statins (which have anti-inflammatory effects) can lower the probability of major depressive disorder.

The observation that many more women than men suffer from major depressive disorder is of interest in the context of both the brain and the immune system. There is a great deal of evidence that the brains of females and males are different. This comes from studies of rodents and nonhuman primates as well as humans, including anatomical and functional imaging, as well as biochemical studies. Of particular relevance for depression are findings of sex differences in the serotonin systems in the brain as well as in the *hypothalamic-pituitary-adrenal axis* (HPA axis, a system that is discussed in the next section). Hormones appear to be involved, since women are at higher risk for depression during periods of hormonal fluctuation—during puberty, in the premenstrual phase, and during and after pregnancy. Rodent studies show that the number and size of synaptic connections between neurons fluctuates during the estrous cycle. In therapy for major depressive disorder, estrogen improves outcomes when administered along with antidepressant medications.

There are also sex differences in the immune system. In rodents, females display stronger antibody responses and greater resistance to foreign grafts than males. In humans, females display higher levels of autoimmune antibodies, and numerous autoimmune diseases occur more frequently in women. Studies of the chronic mild stress model of major depressive disorder (discussed in chapter 6) in rodents have described many responses in the immune system, and these responses show numerous differences between males and females. Moreover, following immune challenge in mice, immune cells taken from males show stronger cytokine responses in the test tube than the cells taken from similarly treated females. Cytokine levels in the blood also vary during the menstrual cycle and during human pregnancy.

The Other Direction: Brain to Immune System Communication

One of the most significant risk factors for major depressive disorder is psychosocial (as opposed to physical) stress. That is, stress in susceptible adults can elicit or exacerbate major depression. In addition, stress during fetal or early childhood development can lead to exaggerated responses to stress in the adult. Such early life events include stress on pregnant women as well as stress on young children. The types of stress that have been studied using epidemiologic methods in this context include experiencing a severe hurricane or losing a spouse during a war. The effects of stress are extremely variable, however, and are influenced by a person's life history, genetic background, and social support network. Work with animals (see box 2.2), where such variables are kept to a minimum, shows that even seemingly very mild stress on newborn rats, such as the mother not licking or grooming them as much as is normal, can have lasting effects. Newborns that do not receive the normal amount of attention end up overreacting to stress as adults. These animals also show signs of depression and anxiety: decreased consumption of sucrose compared to water (less interest in sweets—unlike humans!), less time in open, exposed areas and more time in dark corners, increased startle responses to noises, and a marked increase in consumption of ethanol and even cocaine. Chronic (several weeks) administration of antidepressant agents such as the selective serotonin reuptake inhibitor (SSRI) fluoxetine (Prozac) to adult rats that were maternally deprived as infants/toddlers reverses the state of elevated corticosteroids and heightened anxiety behavior. The SSRI treatment also restores the preference for sucrose and reverses the preference for alcohol. Thus, the depressive-like state induced by stress during early development can be reversed by SSRI treatment in adulthood. The positive response to the medications used in humans suggests that the mechanism of this form of depression in animals resembles that seen in humans.

Box 2.2
Early Life Stress and Adult Anxiety: The Tale of Snowshoe Hares

Why would evolution select for an adult anxiety response to early developmental stress? A suggestion comes from studies of snowshoe hares. The populations of these animals in Canada undergo dramatic increases and decreases
at regular, 10-year intervals (figure 2.2). The large decreases in numbers could

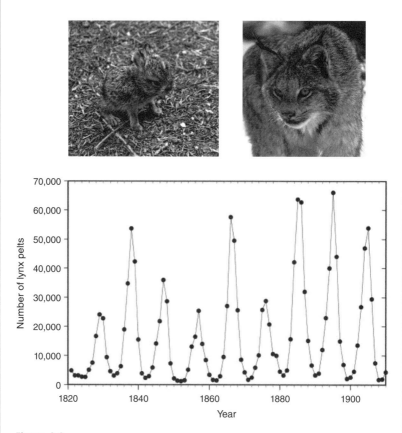

Figure 2.2
Top left: An example of a 12-hour-old snowshoe hare (reprinted with permission from Preisser, *J Animal Ecology*, 78:1103–5, 2009). Right: An example of
a Canada lynx (reprinted with permission from Krebs et al., 2001). Bottom:
Reflecting the fluctuating population of hare predators, the number of Canadian lynx fur pelts sent from the Northern Department of the Hudson's Bay
Company from 1821 to 1910 displays cycles averaging 9.6 years (reprinted
with permission from Elton and Nicholson, *J Animal Ecology* 11:215–44, 1942).
This classic data has subsequently been reproduced by lynx counts in the wild.

Box 2.2
(continued)

be due to decimation of the vegetation when these animals overpopulate, as well as an increase in the population of predators that occurs in response to the abundance of prey. Experiments involving addition of food and exclusion of predators such as lynxes in local habitats indicate that there is an interaction between these two factors, but predation is clearly the dominant process. Other explanations involve cycles of sunspots or conditions related to the North Atlantic Oscillations/El Nino conditions that can affect food resources and the extent of snowfall (which could alter the hunting conditions for predators).

Another factor that is not usually considered in explaining these cycles is the effect of maternal stress. When the number of hares is declining rapidly in the presence of high predator density, each animal is more at risk, as confirmed by higher per capita predation rates during these times. As might be expected, this phase of the cycle is a period of chronic stress, which is evidenced by measurements of elevated blood levels of various stress indicators. Low fecundity has also been measured under these conditions, consistent with increased vigilance and anxiety. Experiments with wild-trapped females show that predator (dog)-induced stress in the laboratory does indeed increase cortisol levels, and it also reduces the size of the offspring. Moreover, females trapped during a period of high stress and taken into the laboratory subsequently maintain low fecundity for an extended period, whereas females taken into the laboratory during a period of low stress maintain high fecundity. This variation represents a long-term change in the physiology of stressed animals. It appears that female hares that were gestating during periods of high stress grow up producing high levels of cortisol, and they are more anxious and likely to be more wary of predators, just like their mothers! The anxiety conferred upon the offspring by their mothers could have an adaptive, beneficial effect on survival, while diminishing the number and/or size of the offspring that the mother produces. This is an example of a maternal influence on the fetus that has direct implications for adult behavior, a topic that will be treated in more detail in the next chapter.

An animal paradigm that has very clear implications for humans involves monkey mothers caring for their infants. In this experiment, one group of mothers received their food in a clearly visible way each day at the front of their enclosure. A second group of mothers had to obtain their food by exploring for the food hidden among wood chips. The third group of mothers had the food presented either visibly (as with the first group) or hidden (as with the second group), but in a random fashion, varying from week to week. Which group exhibited the most stress? The variability in the third setting caused those mothers to show signs of stress, which included mother-infant conflict. The infants, in turn, also exhibited signs of stress, becoming more timid and fearful than the infants in the other groups. Also telling is the observation that the offspring in the third group showed signs of depression, including elevated levels of the peptide CRF in the cerebral spinal fluid, as is seen in human depression. As adolescents, the offspring in the third group were more fearful and submissive, and were involved in less social play. The implications of such animal studies for human infant care are compelling, and provide another example of how stress during early development can lead to a lifelong alteration in mood.

Genetics also play a role. Examination of the effects of stress during early life in humans has revealed that the propensity for major depressive disorder can result from interactions between genetic background and life experiences. For instance, a study by Avshalom Caspi, now at Duke University, and colleagues reported a connection between one variant of the serotonin transporter gene (the short form) and susceptibility to major depressive disorder, including suicidality. This connection requires a history of childhood maltreatment and multiple stressful events in adulthood. People with the long form of the transporter, and with the same life history, are less likely than those with the short form to respond to repeated stressful events in adulthood by becoming very depressed. (Many subsequent studies have replicated this finding, but some have not; although the latter studies have used different methodologies from those in the original work and examined cohorts of people quite different from those in the original report.) One possible explanation for the connection between an early life history of stress and response to stress in adulthood is that the short form of the transporter confers a bias toward negative responses to social stimuli and perceived threats. This is supported by functional magnetic resonance imaging (fMRI) experiments in which people are shown pictures of angry or fearful faces. Those with the short form of the transporter display exaggerated activity in the amygdala, a brain region that responds to social and environmental challenges. They also display increased signs of stress reactivity to such stimuli.

Studies in animal models also support a role for the short form of the transporter in responses to stress. For instance, when infant monkeys are raised among other infants rather than with their mothers, those with the short form display exaggerated stress responses, increased anxiety, and stereotyped, repetitive behaviors compared to the infants with the long form. Similar conclusions were reached using rodent models in which the transporter was genetically manipulated. Interestingly, results from the monkey and rodent experiments further suggest that the effects of the transporter variants on stress reactivity may be due to the role of the transporter in brain development. That is, the activity of the transporter influences the connections that are made between neurons in critical brain areas.

These findings have a number of important implications. First, this transporter is the site at which the SSRI medications act, so its genetic variant could influence the responses to these drugs. Second, since the short form is not rare in human populations, it is not "abnormal" for a person to have this vulnerability. Third, this contribution of genes to psychiatric vulnerability could help to explain why depression can run in families. Fourth, the finding exemplifies the interaction between genes and environment, showing that both factors are critical for a psychiatric condition to manifest itself. Understanding this interaction also helps us see why it has been so difficult to identify genes that enhance vulnerability to disorders such as depression, schizophrenia, and autism. In the retrospective study by Caspi, for example, evoking major depression in people with the short form of the transporter required at least three very significant stressful events earlier in their lives. Most genetic studies at present do not take into account such life events.

But what does psychological stress have to do with the immune system? The brain influences the immune system in several different ways, directly as well as indirectly, via other organs. One direct pathway is from the brain through the sympathetic nervous system into the immune organs—bone marrow, thymus, spleen, and lymph nodes. The sympathetic system is well known for its control of heart rate and blood pressure, and for its role in the fight-or-flight response to danger, preparing the organism for immediate action in the presence of a predator. Part of that evolutionarily appropriate response is to stimulate the *innate* immune system—the part of the immune system that responds very quickly to infection or injury—by sending immune cells to the site, where they can engulf the microbes and kill infected cells with toxins. This is part of the *inflammatory* response, which is also important for wound healing. A ready wound-healing response could also be important with a predator looming. The sympathetic system sends nerves into immune tissues, and immune cells have receptors for the neurotransmitters released by the sympathetic nerves. Neurotransmitters are the small molecules used by neurons to communicate with each other. If blockers of these receptors ("beta blockers") are administered, the effects of acute stressors—the presence of a predator, or giving a public talk, or being asked to solve a difficult problem on the spot—on the immune system are inhibited.

While the innate immune system is activated by acute stress, the other arm of the immune system, the *adaptive* or *humoral* system, is suppressed. The adaptive immune system responds more slowly to environmental challenges, taking time to recognize specific microbes and making antibodies to kill or block them. In the case of an immediate threat or acute stress, resources are shifted away from the adaptive immune system toward the innate immune system.

An interesting example of the sympathetic nerve–immune connection comes from the work of Steve Cole at the University of California at Los Angeles. His group has found a striking effect of chronic stress on the immune system that is mediated by the sympathetic nervous system. Induction of stress in this paradigm involves placing a male monkey in a cage with several other male monkeys that are not part of his normal social group, creating what is known as an unstable social situation. After this is done for 100 minutes daily over 10 months, the density of sympathetic nerves in the lymph nodes doubles (although it is not clear that this actually takes 10 months to occur). The doubling occurs specifically in certain regions of the lymph nodes and does not occur along blood vessels, so it does not represent a general overgrowth of sympathetic nerves everywhere. The growth in the lymph nodes can have significant effects on the response to infection. For instance, replication of the simian immunodeficiency virus, the monkey version of HIV, is much greater in the areas of the lymph nodes adjacent to the sympathetic nerves. This suggests a local effect of the activated nerves on viral infection. That is, it appears that the increase in sympathetic nerves may have resulted in a local increase in viral infection. How might the nerves increase viral load? It is known that chronic stress suppresses the production of the cytokine interferon-beta. Interferon gets its name from its ability to suppress viral replication. Furthermore, activation of sympathetic nerves can inhibit the interferon response to viral infection. Thus, activated sympathetic nerves may allow viral replication by suppressing interferon production. The suggested pathway is: chronic social stress → enhanced sympathetic growth in the lymph node → downregulation of interferon → increased viral replication → disease progression during social stress.

Another, more indirect pathway from the brain to the immune system is also activated by stress. This pathway goes from the cerebral cortex (which perceives the stressful situation), to the hypothalamus (which integrates the information and can regulate appetite, sleep, libido, etc.), to the nearby pituitary gland (which secretes hormones, some of which directly influence immune cells), to the adrenal gland (which secretes several hormones that influence the immune system). This pathway is termed the *hypothalamic-pituitary-adrenal* (HPA) axis (figure 2.3, plate 2). Key hormones secreted by the adrenal gland are cortisol and epinephrine, both of which can act on immune cells. A primary effect of cortisol is to suppress the immune system, which is why it can be used to treat inflammatory disorders such as asthma and rheumatoid arthritis. This effect also helps explain why patients with major depression, who can have elevated cortisol, often display inadequate immune responses.

Cortisol receptors in the brain are part of a feedback loop in which psychological stress activates the HPA axis, leading to increased secretion of cortisol into the blood, which feeds back on the brain, both to activate the hippocampus, a center for learning and memory, and to decrease the number of cortisol receptors. The latter effect protects against excessive cortisol by making the hippocampus less responsive to the hormone. This is important because chronic stress and its associated hormone increases can indeed cause toxic effects on the hippocampus. One such effect is to inhibit the production of new neurons, which is normally ongoing in the adult hippocampus. It is therefore relevant that major depressive disorder

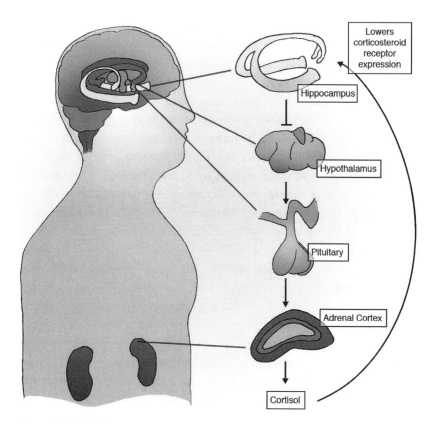

Figure 2.3 (plate 2)
The hypothalamic-pituitary-adrenal (HPA) axis is illustrated, including the feedback of the adrenal hormone cortisol on the hippocampus, where it lowers the level of corticosteroid (cortisol) receptors. (Illustration by Elaine Hsiao)

can involve a faulty cortisol feedback system that renders the hippocampus less effective in its functions. In fact, one of the clinical tests to confirm the presence of major depressive disorder involves measuring HPA axis hormones in the blood following administration of a stressful stimulus.

Patients with major depressive disorder display patterns of immune changes that are similar to those seen with chronic stress, such as blunted antibody responses to vaccination and delayed healing of experimentally administered wounds. Chronic stress, such as with marital discord, loss of a job, or caregiving, is associated with increases in the inflammatory cyto-kine IL-6. If stress persists for extended periods, hippocampal neurons can die. Imaging the brains of patients with posttraumatic stress disorder

(PTSD) using MRI has revealed such atrophy, which could be the result of cell death or inhibition of the normally constant addition of new neurons to the hippocampus. (There is also the possibility that persons susceptible to PTSD have a smaller hippocampus to start with.)

Most of the examples discussed so far involve chronic stress. However, even mild, acute stress affects the immune system. Lymphocytes taken from healthy subjects who underwent a mildly stressful experience, such as speaking in front of a group of volunteers, exhibit elevated markers of inflammation. It is notable that such responses to acute stress are exaggerated in patients with major depressive disorder.

In summary, both experimental animal and human studies indicate that evolution has selected for adaptive responses to acute stress. In the presence of stressful stimuli, the sympathetic nervous system is activated to increase delivery of oxygen and glucose to the heart and skeletal muscle. The innate immune response is activated to enable wound healing and eliminate infection, and the adaptive immune system is turned down. While this is the picture for normal people, patients with major depressive disorder display an exaggerated response to acute stress. Depression also involves symptoms found in people with chronic stress, such as elevated inflammatory cytokines. Elevation of certain cytokines can cause depression, and these proteins are integral to the regulation of the immune response.

The question that began this chapter concerned disease: does the brain influence the immune system to enhance or reduce disease susceptibility? Results from animal studies indicate that the suppression of the immune response that occurs with chronic stress can indeed increase vulnerability to infection and disease. Moreover, in humans, there is evidence that both major depressive disorder and chronic stress are associated with increased susceptibility to a variety of problems such as respiratory infection, cardiovascular disease, and HIV/AIDS. Each of these conditions is known to involve systemic inflammation. An example is the finding that compared to controls, people who score high on measures of psychological stress display exacerbated symptoms and elevated IL-6 responses to an experimental administration of influenza virus. Similarly, the diminished immune function that accompanies normal aging coincides with increased vulnerability to disease and infection.

Animal models have been very effective in probing the effects of stress on the immune system and disease, but they are of little utility in studying the effects of *optimism* on stress. It is difficult to know if a particular manipulation makes a mouse more optimistic! There have been studies in humans, however, that indicate that elevating one's mood while coping with stress can moderate the immunological outcome. Although the link between psychosocial intervention and improvement in cancer outcome remains to be definitively proven, moderating the immune response to the stress caused by a serious illness is likely to be beneficial.

Overall, in this chapter we have seen many examples of how closely intertwined are the immune and nervous systems. These reciprocal interactions occur at many different levels of organization, from the global (hormonal) to the local (synaptic). These interactions are necessary for maintaining homeostasis during a normal, healthy life, and for the response to injury, disease, and negative psychosocial events. In the next chapter we examine immune involvement in embryonic development, which will lead us to the subject of how this immune influence can alter fetal brain development.

3 The Battleground of the Fetal-Maternal Environment

Our mother's wombs the tiring houses be, where we are dressed for this short comedy.
—H. Spenser, "Orlando Gibbons"

The more one learns about the incredible intricacies of the molecular networks involved in embryonic development, the more the word "miracle" comes to mind. For instance, a great deal is being learned about how the layers of cells that make up a developing butterfly's wing work together, in an exceedingly complicated symphony of molecular signals, to construct the highly reproducible pattern of colors in each species. At the same time we are learning that the orchestration of interactions between the fetus, the placenta, and the mother during the development of a human infant is also astounding in its complexity.

At a very early stage, the fetus mounts an inflammatory attack on its mother in order to become established within her, and then the mother's attempt to reject the fetus must be thwarted for it to survive. Given the myriad steps that can go wrong, how is it possible that the vast majority of us turn out so "normal"? In fact, life at these early stages is precarious. The knowledge we are gaining about what can go wrong also helps us understand some of the risk factors associated with faulty fetal brain development that can lead to mental disorders.

Invasion and Colonization of the Mother

First, a few snapshots of early human development: About five days after its fertilization, the egg has become a fluid-filled ball of just 32 cells and has traveled down to the uterus. This ball is called the *blastocyst* (from the

Greek: *blastos*, to sprout or germinate; and *cyst*, cavity), which is about the size of a period on this page. Most important, the blastocyst contains the inner cell mass, which, despite its nondescript name, consists of 12 cells, each of which can, if isolated, develop into a complete human being. These are the famous *stem cells*. However, to survive and develop further, the blastocyst must obtain a blood supply for itself and its stem cells. It does this by attacking the endometrial wall of the uterus, essentially opening up a wound in that tissue, and burrowing into it using enzymes that degrade the endometrium. This is the process of implantation, and this step is the rate-limiting, or weak link in the process of human reproduction. Approximately half of all human embryo implantations fail, ending the pregnancy. Thus, the fate of a pregnancy is often decided at this very early stage. This is also true of in vitro fertilization procedures, which is why multiple blastocysts are injected into the uterus in hopes that at least one will implant successfully.

During this incursion, the cells on the outer layer of the blastocyst develop into invasive, metastasizing cells called trophoblasts (from the Greek: *trephein*, to feed). These cells will eventually populate the placenta, penetrate the uterine blood vessels, and define the border between the mother and the fetus. Thus, trophoblasts mediate the exchange of nutrients into, and waste products out of, the fetus. The trophoblasts also secrete key hormones such as progesterone, which maintain pregnancy. Nonetheless, despite the critical importance of these cells, the mother must eventually stop the invading army of trophoblasts.

The idea that the blastocyst must attack the mother to succeed is supported by experimental evidence from both animals and humans. It was shown more than a hundred years ago that scratching the guinea-pig uterus during an early stage of estrus enhances its receptivity to implantation. In humans, biopsy of the uterus (which produces a local wound) prior to blastocyst injection during the process of in vitro fertilization doubles the success rates for both implantation and live births. Another piece of evidence is that the scar tissue left at the site of previous endometrial surgery or a Cesarean section becomes a preferred site of subsequent implantation.

In fact, high levels of proinflammatory cytokines are produced at the site of implantation. These cytokines are produced by the local endometrial cells as well as by the maternal immune cells that are attracted to the site of implantation. Most of these immune cells are natural killer (NK) cells, which, as their ominous name implies, are used to eliminate cells that are infected with microbes. However, during implantation, NK cells help regulate invasion of the embryo into the uterus, and they secrete angiogenic (from the Greek: *angeion*, vessel) proteins that induce the growth of blood vessels in the forming placenta. Another immune cell that accumulates at the eventual site of implantation, and stays there throughout pregnancy, is the dendritic cell (DC; from the Greek: *dendron*, tree). These highly branched cells are the key initiators of the innate immune response, which rings the first alarm upon recognizing microbes and mobilizes the immune response to fight them. The presence of NK and DC cells at the site of implantation is traditionally thought to be a sign that the mother recognizes a foreign body, the embryo, invading her, and that these cells aid in attempts to eliminate it. This is logical because the embryo does obtain half of its genetic material from its father, which is certainly foreign as far as the mother's immune system is concerned. For instance, if one grafts a piece of the father's skin onto the mother's skin, it will be rejected. (In fact, it is much preferable that the parents be genetically unrelated; witness the problems with the inbred royalty lineages of yore.)

However, new evidence from animal studies indicates that that during pregnancy, DCs are also needed for implantation and for the formation of the placenta. That is, depletion of DCs severely impairs implantation whereas increasing the number of DCs enhances implantation and embryo survival. It has been hypothesized that a high local concentration of DCs in the uterine wall sets up a gradient of inflammatory cytokines, which prepares the endometrium so that the blastocyst can bind there and invade successfully. Part of this preparation may involve local degradation of a web of mucin (a thick mixture of proteins and carbohydrates) that prevents blastocyst adhesion to the endometrium. In this way, the mother initially invites and encourages the incursion.

Thus, the picture of early development is one of an invasion, involving wounding the host and killing cells, with inflammatory signals flaring in abundance, all with essential support provided by maternal immune cells. The result is a complete remodeling of the endometrium at the site of implantation, as the trophoblasts set up a network to commandeer the mother's blood vessels so as to provide nutrients for the embryo. It is perhaps not surprising that during this time the mother experiences morning sickness, possibly because of the proinflammatory state that is set up in her uterus. This state can be even more severe than the usual sickness that is experienced during a cold or a mild case of the flu. It is presently unclear whether the signals that cause nausea during the first trimester resemble any of those sent to the brain during an infection.

This natural proinflammatory state that occurs during early pregnancy must be carefully controlled, as it can be enhanced too much, with dire consequences. For instance, the additional cytokines induced by infection of the reproductive tract can tip the balance toward miscarriage. Thus, there is an optimal level of cytokines that must be maintained at each stage of pregnancy.

The Immunological Paradox of Pregnancy

Once the invasion and colonization of the host mother is successful, a longer, anti-inflammatory phase ensues, during which the mother no longer experiences sickness symptoms and the placenta provides the nutrients, oxygen, hormones, and growth factors needed for rapid fetal growth. The trophoblasts and the maternal immune system also cooperate to fight microbial infection, which may involve bacteria or viruses invading from the vagina or the maternal circulation. But, as previously alluded to, there is also the threat that the maternal immune system will recognize some of the paternal proteins on the fetus as foreign to herself. Since half the genetic contribution to the fetus comes from the father, and the father is normally not genetically related to the mother, the mother will certainly reject those cells displaying proteins from the father. An even more precarious situation is found in donor-egg pregnancies, when eggs from a one woman are fertilized in vitro and the embryos transferred to a gestational carrier. How is the mortal threat to the embryo normally averted?

First, there is evidence that the maternal immune system is altered during pregnancy, but specifically in its response to the foreign signals on the fetus. That is, the mother *tolerates* the foreign body that has invaded her. An animal experiment profoundly illustrates this. A pregnant female mouse will accept and not reject a tumor implanted in her if the tumor is of the same mouse strain as the father of the fetus. That is, if the tumor is genetically closely related to the fetus, the tumor will survive. However, following the birth of her offspring, the mother rejects the tumor. That this temporary immune tolerance is specific is shown by a parallel experiment in which the mother receives a tumor from a mouse strain different from the father of her embryo. She immediately rejects that tumor whether she is pregnant or not. Thus, pregnancy has indeed altered the maternal immune system, but the tolerance is specific for the proteins of the embryo. How is this possible?

One way of inducing this sort of highly specific tolerance involves a special set of immune cells called regulatory T cells, or *Tregs*. These cells are involved in preventing autoimmunity in the adult. That is, if Tregs are depleted, it is easier to produce an immune reaction against one's own cells, and severe autoimmune disease can be initiated early in development. Therefore, it is relevant that the number of Tregs goes up during pregnancy. Conversely, diminished numbers of Tregs are associated with rejection of the fetus. Moreover, the fetuses of miscarriage-prone mice can be protected by injecting the mothers with Tregs. The ability of Tregs to protect is specific to the mouse strain of the fetus. That is, the Tregs of one strain protect the fetus of that strain but not the fetus of another strain. This is consistent with the tumor rejection results just described. But how do the mother's Tregs get "educated" to be able to tone down the mother's immune response specifically to the father's proteins found on the fetus? One theory is that during insemination, the father's sperm evoke a response in the woman that stimulates and "educates" Tregs specifically about his proteins. This is thought to occur in the vagina. Although such a process is still mysterious, one method that is sometimes used to inhibit fetal rejection is vaccination of the prospective mother with proteins from the father's sperm prior to fertilization.

There also appears to be another form of immune suppression during pregnancy, as indicated by the amelioration of symptoms of autoimmune disease such as multiple sclerosis in the mother. One of the mechanisms for this may be the increased level of female hormones that occurs during pregnancy. In fact, a form of estradiol is being tested as a treatment for multiple sclerosis in nonpregnant women. On the other hand, the immune system of the mother does, of course, maintain her ability to fight infection. In addition, the mother passes on her immune capabilities to her offspring. She does this by sending a wide array of antimicrobial antibodies she has acquired during her lifetime through the placenta into the fetus, and also in her colostrum and milk to the newborn. We shall see in chapter

6, however, that if the mother's reaction to an infection is too severe, it can alter fetal brain development and increase the risk for mental disorders such as schizophrenia or autism in the offspring.

A second way of protecting the fetus involves the major histocompatibility complex (MHC) proteins that were discussed in the previous chapter. Recall that MHC proteins on the surface of cells provide key signals used by the immune system to recognize a cell as being foreign. Therefore, it is important that the trophoblasts of the placenta, which provide the first line of defense for the fetus, do not produce certain MHC proteins that could be recognized by the mother's immune cells. Some of these MHC proteins would be inherited from the father, which could lead to killing of these cells by the mother. By not producing these MHC proteins, the trophoblasts in a sense remain immunologically invisible. Interestingly, the same evasion strategy is used by certain pathogens such as the human immunodeficiency virus (HIV). Amazingly, HIV selectively removes certain MHC proteins from the surface of the cells it infects so as to make those cells invisible to potential attacks from the host immune system. It is remarkable that the devious HIV can mimic this clever strategy used by the trophoblasts to protect themselves from the mother's immune system.

Twins, Danger, and Sex

Special problems arise when there are multiple embryos in the uterus. It is therefore of concern that the rate of multiple births is increasing significantly in the United States. This has been attributed to the use of fertility-enhancing drugs and in vitro fertilization. One problem is that, on average, twins are born three weeks early, and significantly premature birth is a major cause of disorders such as cerebral palsy and brain hemorrhage, and there is an increased rate of neonatal mortality as well. These problems are more common in monozygotic (identical) twins, but the mortality risk for dizygotic (nonidentical) twins is 9%, which is still much higher that for singleton births. In fact, the mortality rate for multiple pregnancies is considerably higher than the usually quoted figures of 1% to 3%, because more than 10% of pregnancies begin as multiples but end as singletons when one fetus is lost.

Some particularly dangerous syndromes can occur for twins in utero, especially when the twins share a placenta. It is not widely appreciated

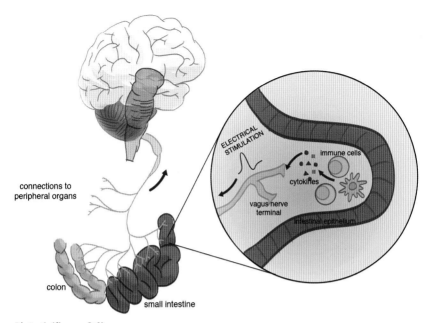

Plate 1 (figure 2.1)
Cytokines evoked by infection, in this case in the gut, stimulate the vagus nerve (yellow) to send electrical signals to the brain. (Illustration by Elaine Hsiao)

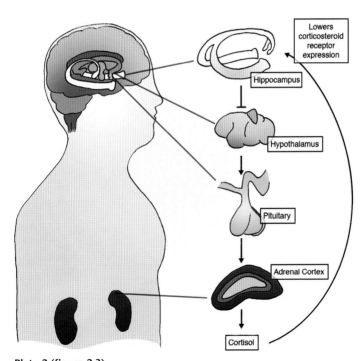

Plate 2 (figure 2.3)
The hypothalamic-pituitary-adrenal (HPA) axis is illustrated, including the feedback of the adrenal hormone cortisol on the hippocampus, where it lowers the level of corticosteroid (cortisol) receptors. (Illustration by Elaine Hsiao)

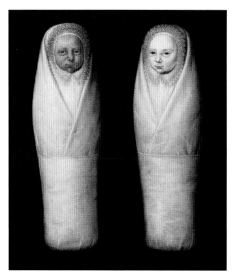

Plate 3 (figure 3.1)
A painting from 1617 known as *de Wikkellkinderen* ("The Swaddled Children") is thought to represent a case of twin-to-twin transfusion syndrome. One of the apparently monozygotic twins appears to be pale and anemic while the other is red and possibly polycythemic (oversupplied with blood). The family history of the owners of the painting suggests that the twins did not survive into adulthood. (Photo from public domain, Wikimedia Commons)

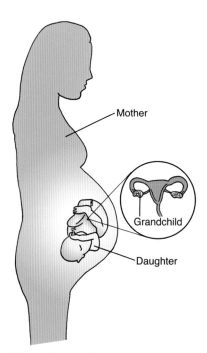

Plate 4 (figure 4.1)
A diagram illustrates the three generations residing in a pregnant female. The future grandchildren are present as eggs in the fetus. (Illustration by Elaine Hsiao)

that about two-thirds of all identical twins share a placenta, which results in competition between them for nutrition. Such twins are significantly lighter at birth than twins who do not share a placenta. One of the dangerous syndromes that can occur with shared placentas is termed the *twin-to-twin transfusion syndrome*; it is the most important risk factor for death or developmental impairment for such twins. In this syndrome one of the embryos diverts much of the blood supply to itself. Even though each embryo has its own region of the single placenta, the nature of the vessels is such that maternal blood flows from one embryo to the other. Depending on the arrangement and size of the blood vessels, the embryo first in line may receive a disproportionate supply of blood, which retards the development of the second twin (figure 3.1, plate 3). Moreover, the embryo first in line can also suffer heart strain due to the unnaturally large volume

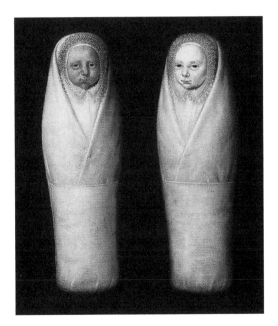

Figure 3.1 (plate 3)
A painting from 1617 known as *de Wikkellkinderen* ("The Swaddled Children") is thought to represent a case of twin-to-twin transfusion syndrome. One of the apparently monozygotic twins appears to be pale and anemic while the other is red and possibly polycythemic (oversupplied with blood). The family history of the owners of the painting suggests that the twins did not survive into adulthood. (Photo from public domain, Wikimedia Commons)

of blood it is forced to pump. Even in the absence of this transfusion pathology, an unequal blood supply is common between monozygotic twins, as is discordant birth weight. As we shall see in the next chapter, a significant difference in birth weight can lead to permanent changes in the physiology of the offspring, including risk of cardiovascular disease and diabetes.

Twin studies are often used to make the point that disorders such as autism and schizophrenia have a very strong genetic component. For instance, in schizophrenia, the concordance for monozygotic twins is 50%. That is, if one twin becomes schizophrenic, the chance that the second twin will develop the disorder is 50%. Since monozygotic twins share identical sets of genes, this high level of concordance is taken as evidence of the importance of the genes in the disease. Dizygotic twins, which do not have identical genes, show a concordance rate of only 17%, and this is seen as further evidence that schizophrenia has a strong genetic basis. However, such conclusions have been criticized for the underlying assumption that monozygotic and dizygotic twins experience the same type of embryonic environments. Since two-thirds of monozygotic twins share a placenta and dizygotic twins never do, the fetal environment is, in fact, quite different for the two classes of twins. That is, the monozygotic twins share an intimate fetal-maternal interface environment as well as genes, whereas dizygotic twins share neither (figure 3.2).

Indirect observations suggest that the concordance for schizophrenia in monozygotic twins that share a placenta is much higher (60%) than in the minority of monozygotic twins that do not share a placenta (11%). This intriguing suggestion needs to be followed up, since it could be very significant in determining the importance of genes in the heritability of schizophrenia. It is also important to note that the concordance for schizophrenia in siblings (from separate pregnancies) is said to be 8%. Since dizygotic twins have the same genetic relatedness as other siblings, it is therefore puzzling why their concordance rate (17%) would be twice as high as that of siblings. One possibility lies in the fact that the dizygotic twins experience the same uterine environment (although not sharing a placenta), while non-twin siblings do not share the same experience during gestation. Thus, on one hand, sharing a placenta should involve the most intimate, common environmental influence. On the other hand, the twin-to-twin transfusion syndrome is an example of how sharing a placenta can

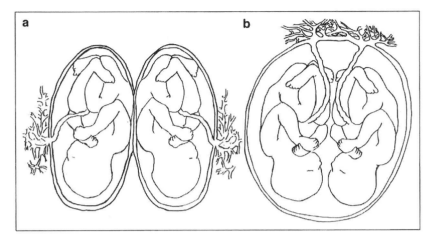

Figure 3.2
Twins can have separate placentas (a) or share one placenta (b) The separate placenta arrangement occurs for all dizygotic twins and for a minority of monozygotic twins. The shared placenta arrangement occurs for the majority of monozygotic twins. (Figure from public domain, Government of South Australia)

lead to very divergent fetal environments. It is clear that for optimal studies of twins and disorders such as schizophrenia, their status with regard to placenta(s) should be taken into account.

Animals that normally carry multiple fetuses, such as rats, mice, and pigs, further demonstrate the importance of sharing (or not sharing) placentas. In these animals the embryos—each with its own placenta—are lined up in the tube-shaped uterus in single file, from the ovary to the vagina. Studies of these multiple fetal-maternal units indicate that each placenta is somewhat different in its ability to transport nutrients and hormones to the fetus. There is additional evidence that the fetal environment can make a significant difference in the physiology and behavior of the fetus. Studies of hormone levels in adjacent embryos indicate that a female embryo positioned between two male embryos has a higher level of testosterone than a female embryo positioned between two female embryos. This suggests that the hormone (or some other sex-specific factor) is diffusing through the placental circulation in levels sufficient to influence nearby embryos. Further support for this idea comes from postnatal observations of the offspring. A female who developed between two males goes on to display more "tomboy-like" behavior than a female that did not have nearby brothers in the womb. The "tomboy" also displays more masculinized anatomical and physiological traits, such as permanently altered hormone levels. This phenomenon has parallels in humans. For instance, a female dizygotic twin with a twin brother displays more risk-taking behavior, is more prone to aggression, and has a more masculine pattern of cerebral lateralization (brain functions assigned to one side of the brain) than a female dizygotic twin with a twin sister. Thus it appears that gender-typical behaviors can be influenced by the embryonic environment as well as by the sex-determination genes.

The same kind of effects could also occur when multiple fetuses with different placentas share the same uterus in the human. For instance, one of the placentas could have a more advantageous or effective placement in the uterine wall, and thus provide better nourishment to its fetus than the other placentas. This could lead to differential susceptibility of the fetus to infection or to the downstream effects of infection, such as the cytokines coming from the mother that fight infection. That is, each individual placenta could filter microbes or cytokines somewhat differently, potentially leading to divergent outcomes for twins with separate placentas. This possibility will be relevant to our discussion of how infection in the mother substantially increases the risk for schizophrenia or autism in her offspring.

A paradox concerning variability among offspring was reported some years ago by Klaus Gartner of the Hannover Medical School in Germany. He studied body weight and the weight of individual tissues such as the kidney in inbred mice housed under laboratory conditions as standardized as possible. Mice that have been inbred for many generations are found to all have the same DNA sequence in their genomes, except for the occasional mutation that crops up. Since they are housed under cage conditions set up to be as controlled and identical as possible, these mice should be as close to exact copies of one another as is possible, for mammals at least. Nonetheless, Gartner found that the body weights for monozygotic co-twins were more similar than for dizygotic co-twins. Monozygotic twins were generated by collecting blastocysts at the eight-cell stage, separating them in half and injecting these four-cell blastocysts into a pseudo-pregnant foster mother. Dizygotic twins were generated by injecting two undivided, eight-cell-stage blastocysts from the same mother into a pseudo-pregnant foster mother. The smaller variance in weights between the monozygotic twins compared to the variance between the dizygotic twins was attributed to a "third component" of development, separate from genetics and environment. At the time this work was done, the nature of the third component was mysterious. Today we postulate that the logical candidate is *epigenetic* modification of the DNA. Epigenetic modification alters the DNA without changing its sequence of bases, which make up the DNA codes for the genes. This modification process, discussed in the next chapter, is also responsible for *genomic imprinting* (see box 3.1). The point

Box 3.1
Battle of the Sexes for Control of the Mind

A strange phenomenon in development called *genomic imprinting* has particular relevance for autism and other disorders that exhibit sexual dimorphism—a preponderance of cases in one sex or the other. During normal development, the fetus inherits one copy of each autosomal (non-sex-linked) gene from each parent. In most cases, RNAs are produced from the genes without regard to the parent of origin. In a minority of cases, however, the gene from one parent is selectively silenced. Most of these imprinted genes are expressed in the placenta or the brain. Since having two functional copies of each gene confers a number of benefits and protections, it is puzzling why some genes are imprinted or silenced according to parent of origin. The leading hypothesis to explain this phenomenon is that it is a consequence of parental conflict over allocation of resources to the offspring, sometimes referred to as the *kinship theory*. By this theory, it is in the father's interest to maximize maternal resources allocated to his offspring. In contrast, it is in the mother's interest to allocate her resources more equitably to her current as well as future offspring, and the latter could come from mating with other males. This theory predicts that paternally expressed genes (for which the copies from the mother are silenced) should be involved in utilizing maternal resources so as to increase the fitness of the fetus. On the other hand, maternally expressed genes (the copies from the father are silenced) should work to oppose the paternally expressed genes. Thus, the imprinted genes are "selfish genes," acting in their own self-interest. This idea is supported by findings that many imprinted genes function in the placenta, in fetal growth, or in suckling behavior.

An example of such selfish genes comes from studies of *insulin-like growth factor 2* (IGF2). In keeping with its name, and with the kinship theory, IGF2 is a paternally expressed gene that stimulates fetal growth. IGF2 exerts its growth-promoting actions by binding to its receptor protein, IGF receptor 1. However, there is also a second IGF receptor (receptor 2), and when IGF binds to this one, IGF is destroyed. As predicted by the kinship theory, the IGF

Box 3.1

(continued)

receptor 2 is maternally expressed. Thus, there is a direct competition between the paternally and maternally controlled genes. Interestingly, while IGF receptor 2 imprinting was initiated during evolution 180 million years ago, it was lost about 75 million years ago with the appearance of primates that gave rise to humans. Thus, while this gene is still imprinted in mice, it is not imprinted in humans (it is, instead, expressed from both maternal and paternal genes). It has been suggested that this change could be due to stable pairing of mates in such primates.

Very recent work from the laboratory of Catherine Dulac at Harvard University has uncovered many new imprinted genes that function in the brain. One of them codes for *interleukin-18*, a cytokine expressed by the maternal gene in the brain, where it can be produced by neurons and by microglial cells. IL-18 has been linked to multiple sclerosis, a disorder that is predominantly found in women. This cytokine has anorexia-like effects in mice, and is elevated in depression, both in patients and in IL-18 animal models. It is also elevated in the serum of schizophrenia patients, as well as in several neurodegenerative diseases and infections of the brain. In fact, a large proportion of the genes that are known to be imprinted are involved in brain disorders.

The relevance of imprinting for autism spectrum disorders (ASD) comes from studies of a cluster of genes on chromosome 15, where there is a hot spot of ASD candidate genes as well as maternal expression. This cluster is disrupted in the disorders known as Angelman syndrome and Prader-Willi syndrome. One of the characteristic features of Angelman syndrome is an unusually positive, happy, and social disposition. This suggests that one of the genes in the cluster on chromosome 15 normally acts as a brake that limits positive social interactions, and that this function is lost when the genes are disrupted. Conversely, patients with Prader-Willi syndrome are prone to depression and temper tantrums. Genetic analysis of Prader-Willi syndrome reveals a double dose of these maternally expressed genes, consistent with an overdose of the braking signals. Abnormalities in this region of chromosome 15 are found in up to 5% of ASD patients, but it remains to be established firmly which of the genes in the cluster are responsible for these various syndromes. It is also unclear what the importance of maternal expression is for these disorders.

These syndromes exemplify the danger of gene imprinting, which is that with only one copy functioning, the effects of a mutation in that copy cannot be compensated for by the other, nonmutant copy of the gene. The mechanism of imprinting involves epigenetic modification of the DNA, a topic that is taken up in the next chapter.

here is that the genetic code itself does not have to be altered in order for the embryos to display differences in development. Nor does the environment surrounding the twins have to be different for the outcome of development to diverge.

Fetal Hormones and Autism

Gender biases the frequency of certain behaviors, and this is likely due to the many structural differences that have been documented between female and male brains. Thus, it may not be surprising that gender can influence disease susceptibility as well. For instance, major depressive disorder, multiple sclerosis, and anorexia are more common in women, while schizophrenia, autism, and attention deficit hyperactivity disorder are more common in males. The incidence of autism, in particular, is four times higher in males than in females.

The autism researcher Simon Baron-Cohen at Cambridge University has postulated that this disorder represents an extreme manifestation of male-typical traits. This idea grows out of his theory of psychological sex differences. It is proposed that, on average, females display a stronger drive to empathize (to identify and respond to others' emotions and thoughts), while males have a stronger drive to systematize (to analyze or construct rule-based systems, such as figuring out how mechanical or natural things work). Consistent with this premise is the finding that autistic subjects score high on systematizing tests but score low on empathizing tests.

Most relevant for this chapter is that these psychological traits correlate with levels of fetal testosterone, which comes primarily from the fetus itself. Testosterone levels can be analyzed from samples taken during normal amniocentesis, because the hormone leaks out of the fetus. When such analysis was done for typically developing children, fetal testosterone levels were positively associated with scores of systematizing and negatively associated with scores of empathizing. This result is consistent with the gender bias in those behaviors. Fetal testosterone levels have also been measured in the case of children who go on to develop autism. Quantification of autistic traits, in such areas as social skills and communication, in those children reveal that the higher the level of fetal testosterone, the more severe the autistic traits. This correlation holds for children of both sexes, suggesting that the traits represent an effect of the hormone and not just the sex of the child. This result supports the hypothesis that elevated testosterone can influence fetal brain development in such a way as to predispose to autistic traits. Since testosterone has many important effects on brain development, sorting out which effect is related to these behaviors will not be easy. Work with animal models that display autistic-like traits will be useful in this regard. Such models are discussed in chapter 6.

In this chapter we have briefly reviewed embryonic development, with an emphasis on the involvement of immune cells and proteins. We have also begun to explore some of the factors that influence fetal brain development in ways that increase the risk for mental illness. In chapter 4 we review embryonic development using the framework of "fetal programming"—preparing the fetus for life outside the womb—and explore how such programming can lead to disease in the adult.

4 Prenatal Origins of Adult Health and Disease

Is life worth living? This is a question for an embryo not for a man.
—Samuel Butler

Nothing happens to anybody which he is not fitted by nature to bear.
—Marcus Aurelius Antonius

Fetal Programming

We learned in the previous chapter of the embryo's struggle to implant successfully, to fend off rejection by the mother and, in some cases, to compete for resources with another embryo in the same womb. The environment experienced by the fetus during its further development in the mother's body can also have lifelong effects on its health. As we shall see, aspects of the fetal environment can help determine the risk for future adult disorders such as cardiovascular disease, stroke, osteoporosis, certain cancers, asthma, and diabetes, as well as depression and schizophrenia. The term *fetal programming* is often used to refer to the capacity of the mother to influence the lifelong health outcome of her offspring during its gestation. This phrase is perhaps too deterministic: the fetal environment can set the level of risk, but the embryo's genes also play a role, as does the postnatal environment. Nonetheless, the mother's influence during gestation on the eventual health of her adult offspring is considerable.

The notion that adult disease is influenced by the environment experienced by the developing fetus was highlighted by the early work of the British epidemiologist David Barker (see box 4.1). Barker was struck by some surprising and intriguing findings regarding birth weight and disease. In the birth records of early twentieth-century England, he found that

Box 4.1
David Barker

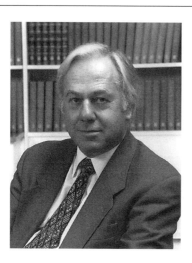

David Barker received his MD from Guy's Hospital in London and then did graduate work in epidemiology at the University of Birmingham. In 1972, he joined the faculty at the new medical school being constructed in Southampton. Away from London, Cambridge, and Oxford, this location was perhaps appropriate for Barker's outsider status as he put forth the decidedly anti-establishment "Barker hypothesis." His data supporting the idea that the fetal environment can influence the risk for heart disease, hypertension, stroke, obesity, osteoporosis, and breast cancer was seen as a direct challenge to the prevailing medical view that "heart disease is your own fault," as Barker puts it. Many feared that an emphasis on the role of the pregnant woman's health and nutritional status in the adult health outcome of her fetus would undermine public health measures to warn about poor lifestyle choices in adulthood, which can indeed influence heart disease risk. In fact, the data that Barker and many others have collected around the world indicate that the fetal environment is likely to set the level of a person's susceptibility to the risks posed by subsequent lifestyle choices.

Barker is currently also a professor at the Oregon Health and Science University in Portland, where he and his colleagues are continuing the effort to illuminate the critical role of the mother's health status on the health outcome of her offspring, and also on the disease risk for her daughters' daughters—her grandchildren. Variety in the maternal diet is key, and being too thin or too fat during pregnancy are warning signs for the offspring.

Box 4.1
(continued)

> However, Barker admits that changing food choices and diet will require a cultural shift regarding eating and cooking. He also rails against the current dominance of genetics research in the funding of biomedical science. Nonetheless, the Barker hypothesis seems to have finally gone mainstream, as illustrated by the title of a recent paper from Harvard, "The Fetal Origins of Adult Disease: From Skeptic to Convert." (Photo courtesy of D. Barker)

being born small for one's gestational age carries increased risk for cardiovascular disease in adulthood. For both men and women, the risk of eventual death from heart disease in people born weighing less than 5.5 pounds is twice as high as that for people born weighing more than 9.5 pounds. The increased risk was found to be graded across all birth weights. That is, the risk associated with being small for one's age at birth does not just apply to the smallest, premature babies. Rather, it forms a continuum across all healthy babies—low risk at higher birth weights and high risk at lower birth weights.

The effect remains even after taking into account postnatal lifestyle factors of the offspring such as exercise, diet, and socioeconomic status. While such factors are indeed relevant to the risk of heart disease, so is birth weight. Similar findings have been made around the world. For instance, in a study of 100,000 American nurses, blood pressure in adulthood could be predicted by weight at birth! Moreover, low birth weight is also associated with increased risk for type 2 (formerly called adult-onset) diabetes. Type 2 diabetes is associated with hypertension as well as cardiovascular disease, and this cluster of problems is termed the metabolic syndrome.

Interestingly, a new epidemiologic study covering 1.49 million people in Sweden and Denmark showed that schizophrenia risk is associated with low birth weight. Moreover, as in the metabolic syndrome, there is a linear relationship for schizophrenia risk across all birth weights—the lower the weight, the higher the risk, but the risk is not confined to just the very smallest babies. This association is also true for global cognitive ability measured at ages 6 to 8 years, in adolescence, and into adulthood.

What came to be known as the Barker hypothesis can be framed in the context of evolution. The idea is that the fetus adapts to the gestational environment provided by the mother. If she is suffering nutritional deprivation, the deprived fetus limits its growth to conserve the resources available to it in order to survive to birth. In fact, being born smaller than normal would also be an advantage in the mother's world of scarce food resources; the offspring would require less food to sustain itself. This "thrifty phenotype" notion provides an evolution-based explanation for the observation that thin or small mothers tend to give birth to smaller babies. In addition, thin female offspring also tend to have an earlier onset of puberty, which, in a world of diminished resources and increased competition, may enhance the family's chances of survival if reproduction occurs earlier in life, before the female becomes unhealthy or loses out in the competition for food. The nutritional status of the mother also influences the size and dimensions of the placenta, and these measurements turn out to be excellent predictors of disease in the adult offspring. The findings about the placenta appear to reflect its crucial role in providing both nutrients and hormones to the fetus, and its function in translating the nutritional and hormonal status of the mother to the fetus.

Genes are also important in the risks associated with low birth weight. There are several types of dopamine receptors in the brain. These receptors are the proteins that bind the neurotransmitter dopamine, which is critical for many types of behavior: responses to rewards such as food and sex, and the related phenomenon of addiction; movement and the lack of it in Parkinson's disease; learning and cognition. The gene for one of these dopamine receptors comes in several versions in human populations. In a study of cognition that is similar to the Wisconsin Card Sorting test that will be discussed in the context of schizophrenia in chapter 6, it was found that a cognitive deficit was present in people who had one particular version of this dopamine receptor gene. However, just having the gene variant was not enough to cause the deficit—it had to be coupled with low birth weight. That is, having the gene variant did not cause the deficit in individuals of normal birth weight. Moreover, low birth weight itself was not associated with the cognitive deficit; one had to also have the gene variant. This is an example of what is called gene-environment or GxE interaction. Simply knowing the DNA sequence of this gene is not enough to predict performance on the cognitive test. The influence of the gene is dependent on the context—in this case, likely the nutritional status of the mother, during and probably before pregnancy.

There are many reasons babies are born at a lower weight than normal. These include having a twin, having a genetic growth disorder, and gestating in a malnourished mother. A classic illustration of the latter concerns a seven-month period during the Second World War in the Netherlands. During this time, often termed the Dutch Hunger Winter, the Nazis imposed severe food rationing on the country as punishment for the resistance to the German occupation. Despite the dire conditions, Dutch hospitals continued to keep careful records of pregnancies and births. Women who were pregnant during this period gave birth to smaller babies on average, and the babies gestating during this Hunger Winter went on to develop higher rates of obesity and insulin resistance. In addition, these offspring developed schizophrenia at a higher rate than offspring gestating before or after the famine. We shall return to the maternal risks associated with schizophrenia in chapter 5, and discuss ideas about how these risk factors might impact fetal brain development to cause mental illness.

The Dutch famine also had a transgenerational effect: grandchildren of the women who were pregnant during the Hunger Winter also turned out to be smaller than average at birth. Perhaps this should not be surprising in light of the fact that these grandchildren came from eggs that were developing in the fetuses gestating during the famine! (See figure 4.1, plate 4.)

Mismatch in Prenatal versus Postnatal Environments

If the postnatal environment does not match that which was predicted by the signals received by the fetus during gestation, the mismatch can increase the risk for adult onset disease. This is shown most clearly in animal studies. Studies with rats, sheep, and other animals have found that reducing caloric intake during pregnancy, or lowering the protein content, but then feeding the offspring a normal diet postnatally yields adults with hypertension. These offspring also have a shorter life span. They can also display an increased response to stress as adults; that is, they are less resistant to the effects of stress. The mismatch hypothesis is further supported by other types of diet reversal experiments. Rats exposed to a high-fat diet during gestation and then given a normal postnatal diet develop blood-vessel pathology, while those that are exposed to the high-fat diet during

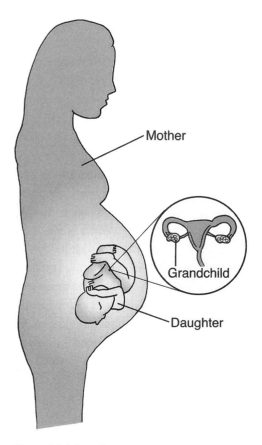

Figure 4.1 (plate 4)
A diagram illustrates the three generations residing in a pregnant female. The future grandchildren are present as eggs in the fetus. (Illustration by Elaine Hsiao)

gestation and then continue with such a diet postnatally do not have this problem.

Also consistent with the mismatch notion is evidence from third-world countries that are beginning to experience a Western diet. The incidence of noncommunicable diseases such as cardiovascular pathology and diabetes is rising in those countries. How do we know that this has anything to do with a pre- and postnatal mismatch? Studies suggest that the risk is highest in the offspring of poorly nourished women. The "thrifty phenotype" in which the postnatal offspring of nutritionally-deprived mothers display increased appetite and increased storage of energy as well as decreased energy expenditure, will promote obesity.

Obesity, Depression, and Inflammation

Obesity is not only increasing in underdeveloped countries; it is said to now be at epidemic levels in both children and adults in the United States. Although the number of fat cells (adipocytes) is set during childhood (or before), the amount of fat stored in each cell can increase dramatically in response to diet. Why is obesity a topic of interest for a book on neuroimmune interactions? It is clear that increased adipose tissue in the abdomen activates the innate immune system—the part of the immune system that responds immediately to microbes, and components of which are found in the brain. Moreover, lipid accumulation in adipocytes stimulates the adipose tissue to secrete inflammatory cytokines such as IL-6. Also secreted are chemoattractant proteins that attract cells such as lymphocytes from the immune system into the fat deposits. Thus, increased lipid accumulation results in a chronic inflammatory state, particularly in the abdomen. The increase in inflammatory cytokines can also affect behavior, as we have discussed previously. Of particular relevance is a connection with major depressive disorder. Many (but not all) studies have shown that obesity increases the risk for depression, and that prior depression increases the risk for obesity. In particular, excess visceral (abdominal) fat is associated with the onset of depression. Consistent with these findings are studies showing that people who consume high levels of fish or fish oil display low levels of major depressive disorder. Moreover, even a small increase in fish intake is associated with reduced depression severity. The general health benefits of fish and fish oil consumption may occur through several mechanisms, but a major factor is likely to be a reduction in the inflammatory state.

Given that the rates of obesity, depression, and suicide have increased not only in adults but in children and adolescents, it is natural to ask whether similar interrelationships between these factors play out in children as well as in adults. In fact, childhood depression predicts both adult depression and the type of metabolic disorders associated with obesity. One encouraging bit of data in this otherwise dark picture comes from a small study of dietary intervention in depressed children. In a placebo-controlled experiment with children at high risk for depression, only 12 weeks of dietary intervention provided protection for at least 40 weeks.

How are depression, obesity, and inflammation related? Which influences which? One model suggests a causal pathway leading from depression to adiposity to inflammation and elevated cytokines such as IL-6. However, since obesity can have a negative impact on self-esteem, the pathway could run in the reverse direction. In addition, major depressive disorder influences eating behavior and physical activity, which suggests a more complex, reciprocal relationship between depression, obesity, and the proinflammatory state. For instance, sustained exercise in both adults and children reduces markers of inflammation. Recall also from chapter 2 that inflammatory disorders such as multiple sclerosis, psoriasis, and cardiovascular disease are associated with depression. Moreover, depression often involves increases in circulating cytokines such as IL-6, and injection of certain cytokines can induce depression. In addition, certain anti-inflammatory drugs can decrease symptoms of depression. The sum of these observations suggests a complex, reciprocal set of interactions between inflammation, obesity, and depression.

A new twist to this story involves viral infection and obesity. Although adenoviruses can cause respiratory infections, infection with a different type of adenovirus can increase body fat in rodents, chickens, and non-human primates. Moreover, studies both in adults and in children have found that this virus is three times more common in obese individuals than in controls. In addition, the vast majority of obese children tested positive for antibodies against the virus, indicating a recent or current infection. Among obese children, those that are positive for the virus are significantly heavier than those that are negative for the virus. Although it is not yet clear how the virus is connected to body weight, one finding in animals is that this virus alters the synapses in the hypothalamus, a brain area that controls feeding behavior and metabolism. On the other hand, since obesity alters immune function, it is also possible that obese people are more vulnerable to this type of viral infection. In any case, this research on adenoviruses demonstrates another connection between the immune system and obesity, with significant public health implications.

Epigenetics

In fetal programming, how does the maternal environment in the womb influence the health outcome for the fetus in adulthood? It is very unlikely that the actual sequence of bases in the DNA of the fetus is altered. That is, the adult offspring should have the same set of genes that it had as a fetus. However, during normal development there are numerous changes in the pattern of *expression* of the genes—that is, in the set of genes that is "turned on" to make RNA and then protein, and the set that is "turned off" and silenced. For instance, some of the genes that are needed for early fetal brain development are strongly turned on during that period, but may not be needed in adulthood, and so are turned off. Gene expression can also be tissue specific: although all cells in the body contain the same set of genes, some of the genes that are expressed during brain development may not be expressed in the developing heart. This seemingly miraculous variety is all part of normal, otherwise unremarkable embryonic development.

The expression of genes can be regulated in a number of ways. One of the molecular mechanisms that has only recently come to be widely appreciated is termed *epigenetic* (from the Greek: *epi*, above, over). We will use this term to refer to changes to the genome that do not involve altering the DNA sequence, but which are inherited by daughter cells after they have divided. That is, it is possible to change the *expression* of genes, permanently or semipermanently, without changing the sequence of the DNA itself. This can be done, for instance, by biochemically adding modifying groups to the bases in the DNA. An example of this is *methylation*. Methylation is one of several ways to silence genes, keeping them from producing RNA and eventually protein. Adding a methyl group to a region of the DNA that codes for a certain gene makes it more difficult for that gene to be expressed as RNA.

Silencing genes can be good or bad. It is important that some genes be turned off or turned down. The genes that are responsible for making the proteins of the lens in the eye must be controlled appropriately or this structure would become too thick to see through. Conversely, if those same genes are not turned on at the correct time during development, we would not have a lens to focus the light on the retina.

The Epigenetic Archive of Prenatal Conditions

We now know that epigenetic regulation of gene expression through methylation occurs in the context of maternal-fetal interaction. A classic example involves folic acid. If a woman does not eat enough folic acid during early pregnancy, the baby may be born with defects of the neural tube, the precursor to the brain and spinal cord. One of the functions of folic acid is to aid in DNA methylation, and animal studies have shown that changing the level of folic acid in the diet can alter the methylation, and hence the expression, of particular genes. In one strain of mice, for instance, folic acid supplementation of an otherwise nutritionally adequate diet during pregnancy permanently changes the coat color of the offspring. It does this by altering the expression of a gene involved in determining coat color. It is worth noting that this result raises a question about what unexpected side effects may be occurring in our modern diet of folic acid–supplemented foods. While this diet is credited with lowering the frequency of neural tube defects, one wonders what other effects it may be having on gene expression.

Another demonstration of the effect of the maternal environment on the epigenetic state of the fetus comes from studies of the offspring of women who were pregnant during the Dutch Hunger Winter. Blood samples were recently taken from these offspring, now over 60 years of age, and the methylation state of a number of genes of interest was analyzed. Indeed, in parallel to the findings of animal studies, maternal malnutrition around the time of conception caused a small but significant change in the methylation of certain genes that are known to be important in human growth and development. Moreover, the methylation state of at least one of those genes is known to be affected by maternal folic acid supplementation. Some of the affected genes were more methylated while others were less methylated than in siblings born just before or after the Hunger Winter. It follows, then, that some genes are more likely to be turned on while others are more likely turned off in the offspring of women who were pregnant during the Hunger Winter, in comparison to people who did not experience that deprived prenatal environment.

The results from the Dutch Hunger Winter study, coupled with animal studies, indicate that epigenetic changes in the fetus that were driven by the maternal environment can be permanent. There is also evidence that some epigenetic changes are heritable across generations.

One of the documented risk factors for schizophrenia is being born to a mother who experienced severe stress during pregnancy. Examples of such stress that have been studied include death of the father during gestation or the mother undergoing a life-threatening experience. To understand how this risk factor works, animal models are being studied. Such experiments have defined various factors that can influence the outcome of maternal stress and even described structural changes in the brains of the offspring. Some of the effects of maternal stress have been found to continue beyond the adult offspring, extending to the second generation of progeny. The animal studies have also provided insights into the mechanisms that mediate both the effects of maternal stress on the fetus and the resulting behavioral abnormalities in adult offspring. Some of these behaviors are analogous to those seen in human major depressive disorder or schizophrenia.

These findings are relevant in the present context because methylation is involved in the fetal response to maternal stress. Moreover, the placenta plays a role in mediating the chain of events. An enzyme that is important in maintaining DNA methylation is significantly lower in male placentas of stressed mothers compared to female placentas of those same mothers. This suggests that female placentas may be better able to maintain methylation under stress. In addition, there are methylation changes in the fetal brain itself. In the hippocampus, a region required for learning, the methylation and expression levels of the cortisol receptor are altered by maternal stress in a sex-specific manner. This is important because cortisol levels are sharply increased by stress, and elevation of cortisol for significant periods of time can damage the hippocampus. Increases in the cortisol receptor, the protein that recognizes and binds this hormone, can exacerbate the detrimental effects of the hormone in the brain.

Another case of epigenetic control involving the cortisol receptor concerns the level of care that a mother gives her newborn offspring. A series of studies on maternal care in rats by Michael Meaney, Moshe Szyf, and their colleagues at McGill University in Montreal showed that the offspring of mothers who actively lick and groom their newborn pups grow up to display lower levels of reaction to stress as adults compared to offspring of mothers who are deficient in such maternal care. Both sets of pups grow up, leave home, as it were, and don't call or write, but the offspring who experienced less nurturing care are less able to handle stress as adults. More frightening still, when these offspring give birth to pups themselves, they too display low levels of maternal care. This transgenerational effect has also been observed in studies of nonhuman primates.

How do we know this trait is not being transmitted via the sequence of the DNA in the genes of the mothers? Experiments using a cross-fostering paradigm are used to make the distinction. In this type of study, the pups born to a mother who is deficient in maternal care are transferred at birth to a mother known to show a high level of maternal care. These pups grow up to display normal reactions to stress rather than hyper-responsiveness. In the converse experiment, when pups newly born to a high maternal care mother are transferred to a low maternal care mother, they grow up to be hyperresponsive to stress and, as adults, go on to display low levels of maternal care to their own offspring. How is this series of behavioral traits transmitted across generations? The cross-fostering experiment shows that the traits are not carried by the DNA sequence of the *genes* of the mothers, but rather by the *environmental* influence of maternal care. In a further direct, but exhausting experiment, the research-ers could mimic the effects of good maternal care by stroking the pups with a brush.

Meaney, Szyf, and colleagues went on to show that the gene for the cortisol receptor in the hippocampus of the offspring is methylated to dif-ferent extents in the pups that receive high versus low maternal care. Low maternal care results in more methylation, which prevents normal expres-sion of the receptor. This differential methylation is likely to be responsible for the difference in adult stress responsivity. For instance, when they experimentally manipulated the methylation of the gene for the cortisol receptor by using a chemical that alters the activity of enzymes responsible for methylation, the researchers were able to reverse the effects of low maternal care. That is, they infused a chemical that removed methyl groups from the cortisol receptor in the adult offspring of low maternal care mothers. This resulted in increased levels of the cortisol receptor, and in turn, reversed the hyperresponsivity of these offspring to acute stress. Thus, the epigenetic change to the DNA methylation of the cortisol recep-tor affects the stress responses in the adult offspring, and this methylation is influenced by maternal care. The fact that normal responses to acute stress can be restored in the adult offspring indicates that the effects of low maternal care can be reversed, which offers hope for future treatment strategies in humans who experienced severe stress in early life.

It should be mentioned, however, that some experts in the field of epigenetics are not quite ready to accept this entire story. They point out that there are several gaps in our knowledge regarding how methyl groups are actually removed from the DNA, and that the changes in methylation status are quite small. Nonetheless, similar correlations of methylation status with behavioral experience are continuing to appear in the scientific literature.

It may seem that the effects of maternal care in the rat model have obvious implications for the human response to early life stress, but it is important to determine just how much of this work on rats really does carry over to humans. Recent studies have compared post-mortem brains from suicide victims to the brains of individuals who died of other sudden causes (auto accidents, etc.). Suicide victim tissue was used for the purpose of examining the physiologic influence of psychiatric status. The investigators also examined the life histories of all subjects in the study. One finding was that a developmental history of childhood mistreatment predicts the altered DNA methylation status of the cortisol receptor gene in the hippocampus. This finding appears to be relevant to the issue of maternal care and consistent with the maternal care data for rats.

A second result was that the samples from suicide victims showed more methylation at the cortisol receptor site than did the samples from control (non-suicide) subjects, similar to what is seen in the offspring of animals providing low maternal care. However, the methylation increase in the suicide victims' brains was apparent only if the subject also had a history of childhood mistreatment. These results are consistent with the idea that variations in maternal care can influence the epigenetic state of a part of the human genome that is important in stress responsivity and immune suppression. They also support the link between childhood abuse and increased stress response in adult humans.

Other recent observations have linked DNA methylation with psychiatric conditions. One such condition is Rett syndrome (RTT; see text box 4.2). This is a progressive neurodevelopmental disorder that occurs predominantly in girls. Although its symptoms vary considerably, RTT is one of the most common causes of mental retardation in females. Rett syndrome can also be accompanied by autistic symptoms. The key point here is that RTT is caused by mutations in a gene that codes for a protein (MeCp2) that binds methylated DNA. MeCp2 regulates the expression of

Box 4.2
Falling Silent

After a child is born, parents watch with anticipation the normal developmental program that ensues. The baby smiles and follows faces at 6 weeks, acquires sufficient motor control to sit and transfer toys by 6 months, and typically walks and says a couple of words by 12 to 15 months. Language and thought continue to develop as children begin to understand make-believe play, to use verbs to describe a mental state, and to imitate complex actions.

Ashley delighted her parents as she progressed through early developmental milestones. She learned to crawl, babble, walk, and sing nursery rhymes, all at the expected ages. At 18 months, however, her progress ceased. No more songs or words, only a vacant stare. Ashley's ability—or inclination—to use her hands was overwhelmed by incessant hand-wringing; tremors, rocking, and loss of balance robbed her of normal motor control; apnea and hyperventilation indicated autonomic control was going haywire, too. Her head growth slowed, and her social interactions became almost nonexistent.

Alex, born to a different family at a different time, has a similar story. He was a healthy boy who smiled and followed faces by 6 weeks, made eye contact, and enjoyed interactive games. At 10 months of age he showed an unusually intense interest in wheels, but he continued to interact socially and was saying several words and walking by 13 months. Sometime between 15 and 18 months, however, Alex, like Ashley, fell silent. He stopped trying to communicate through gestures or words. He lost interest in social interactions and became utterly absorbed with lines on a tile or wheels on a toy. He seemed less sensitive to pain but hypersensitive to heat. He flapped his hands constantly and picked at his skin.

Similar histories, different diagnoses: Ashley has Rett syndrome and Alex has autism. Both disorders become manifest after a period of apparently normal development. Both disrupt social and language development and are accompanied by unusual stereotypies. Despite the intellectual regression that marks the majority of Rett patients and approximately 30% of autistic patients, neither disease is neurodegenerative in nature. Many children can improve somewhat as they get older. Although neither Ashley nor Alex have any language skills, they do have better eye contact now and seem to recognize family and friends at their respective ages of 23 and 11 years. (Excerpted from Zoghbi, 2003.)

many genes in the brain, and so has far reaching effects on brain function. Thus, RTT provides a classic case of the importance of DNA methylation in brain development.

The fact that DNA methylation, while stable, can be reversed postnatally provides hope for disorders such as RTT, as discussed in chapter 9.

Social and Economic Implications

As we saw in chapter 1, Douglas Almond showed that, on average, the offspring of women who were gestating at the time that the 1918 Spanish flu came through their area grew up to have lower income, socioeconomic status, and educational attainment than those gestating just before or after the pandemic. This finding, combined with previous findings on the long-term health effects of the prenatal period, helps explain the connection between adult health and economic outcomes (see box 4.3). In his article, Almond concludes,

That fetal health may be at the fulcrum of this relationship suffers no shortage of policy implications. The most pressing among these concerns racial disparities in the United States. Early-life health measures of blacks have stagnated since the late 1990s: a black infant is currently more than twice as likely to die before age 1 as a white infant. The results of this [Almond's] study indicate that a future of racial inequality is being programmed. Interventions targeting early-life health of black infants hold promise for reducing racial disparities in adult health and economic outcomes. Identifying efficient public policies to achieve this end should be a priority of future research.

In this chapter we have briefly reviewed some issues of fetal brain development using the framework of fetal programming as a vehicle for discussion. It is clear that a mother's behavior and mental state can influence fetal development and even the eventual health of the adult offspring. These influences go well beyond maternal use of drugs of abuse to include factors that can be out of the mother's control, such as stressful events or lack of food. It is also important to realize that these changes in fetal brain development can, at least in some cases, be passed on to a subsequent generation beyond the fetus in question. We also discussed new information on the molecular mechanisms that help to explain how these physical and mental traits are passed down through the generations. The next chapter examines a different influence on fetal outcome: maternal infection.

Box 4.3
Epigenetic Epilogue: The Tragic Case of the Midwife Toad

In the early twentieth century, the field of biology was one of active discovery and theorizing as well as controversy. Mendel's laws of genetics were coming to be appreciated even though an understanding of the molecular nature of genes was still a long way off. The mechanisms underlying Darwinian evolution were being hotly debated, and the eugenics movement, favoring selection of the "best" people for propagation and gradual elimination of the less desirable, was very active. Jean-Baptiste Lamarck's name became the one most prominently attached to the idea of the inheritance of acquired traits. An oft-cited example is the long necks of giraffes, which were said to result from reaching up for leaves high in trees. This reaching stretched the neck, and the longer necks were passed down to the generations that followed. Heritability of acquired traits might also mean that improvement in one's athletic ability or musical talents, for instance, could be passed on to one's offspring. Although Darwin had favorably speculated about variations brought on by environmental pressures being inherited, he was not able to offer a useful explanation for how this might occur. Mendelian genetics, on the other hand, did suggest a mechanism for natural selection, which led eventually to discarding the theory often termed "Lamarckism."

Despite this environment, in 1926 a young and charismatic popularizer of biological ideas, Paul Kammerer, published a book entitled *The Inheritance of Acquired Traits*. Kammerer's vision was that man could control his own evolution in a positive way. He promoted a "creative" type of evolution rather than one that worked by elimination through natural selection. Thus, intellectual progress and innovation in the arts would accumulate by inheritance, and human evolution would continue in a positive direction. Working as an assistant in the private "Institute for Experimental Biology" that was built in an amusement park outside of Vienna, Kammerer found what he felt was convincing evidence that the changes he produced in a variety of animals by experimentally altering their environments could be inherited.

The most famous example involved the midwife toad (see figure 4.2). This unusual amphibian lives and mates on land, and the male takes the eggs from the female and attaches them to his hind legs for safe incubation. Thus, the eggs develop out in the air, and they are delivered to the water only later, at the tadpole stage. In related species of aquatic toads, in contrast, copulation occurs in the water and males develop specialized structures on their forelimbs, called nuptial pads, during the mating season. These are pigmented and rough, which aids the male in grasping the slippery female during mating. Importantly, the terrestrial midwife toad lacks these pads.

Kammerer did an experiment in which he raised the midwife toads in unusually warm and dry conditions. In this environment, these normally

Box 4.3
(continued)

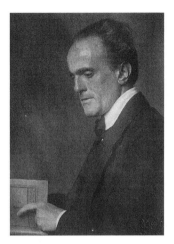 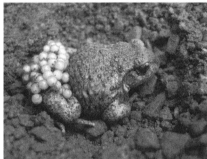

Figure 4.2
Left, Paul Kammerer (photo from Library of Congress); right, a male midwife toad carrying eggs. (Photo courtesy of Simon Beignier)

terrestrial animals spent most of their time in basins of cool water, where they copulated. The eggs so produced then developed in the water and, like aquatic toads, were not carried by the male. While only a few of these eggs went on to complete development, those animals that survived to adulthood were reported to copulate in the water and release their eggs there, even under normal ambient temperature conditions. Thus, they behaved like aquatic toads. Kammerer said that these water-preferring toads bred true, in the sense that they maintained this acquired characteristic of preferring the aquatic lifestyle, through six generations. He also reported that by the fourth generation, these toads started to develop the nuptial pads normally seen in aquatic toads. In addition, Kammerer cross-bred some of the original midwife toads with the new toad variants and reported "Mendelian" proportions of "land" versus "water" toads among the offspring. He therefore argued that these inherited characteristics followed the genetic rules laid down by Mendel.

These very striking findings were not accepted by most of the contemporary scientists who were engaged in debates about the mechanism underlying Darwinian evolution. Part of the problem was clearly Kammerer's mixed Jewish heritage and German anti-Semitism. Another issue was his flashy style and his exuberant lectures and claims. He had a high profile in the popular press and was very much a part of fin-de-siècle Vienna high

Box 4.3
(continued)

society. He socialized with his idol Gustav Mahler, and had a serious affair with Mahler's famously amorous wife Alma. She apparently was the stimulus for a Kammerer treatise on the inheritance of musical talent in the evolution of the arts. He even convinced her at one point to work in the laboratory on praying mantises. Kammerer was so passionate about Alma that he repeatedly threatened suicide, waving a gun in front of her, unless she married him.

Another, more serious problem in convincing his contemporaries of his theories was Kammerer's failure to carefully document his findings. The illustrations and photographs of his animals were poor, and they did not clearly support his claims. The dénouement came in 1926, when the professional herpetologist G. Kingsley Noble examined the last remaining living example in Kammerer's collection of the "aquatic" version of the midwife toad and found that the pigment spot in the supposed nuptial pad had been made by injection of India ink. Noble published this evidence of apparent fraud, and shortly thereafter Kammerer shot himself on a mountain trail outside Vienna.

The decades following his suicide have seen much debate as to the veracity of Kammerer's claims for the inheritance of acquired characteristics. Unfortunately, no one has published experiments attempting to replicate his findings with midwife toads. However, with the new science of epigenetics, we now know that environmental manipulations can indeed alter DNA, as in the case of maternal care and methylation, and that such alterations in the genes can be inherited in some cases. Moreover, recent scrutiny of the details of Kammerer's findings has raised the possibility that his midwife toad experiment could be the first reported case of epigenesis, although there is no molecular documentation to support it. If it could be shown that his experiments did involve DNA methylation, Paul Kammerer, rather than being a tragic fraud, could be seen as the unwitting discoverer of epigenetics.

5 Infections and Behavior

And time future contained in time past.
—T. S. Eliot, "Burnt Norton"

Adult Infections and Behavior

For decades, suspicions have been voiced in the medical literature about potential connections between infectious agents, particularly viruses, and schizophrenia. Some of the suspicion, especially in the past, was due to the mysterious nature of viruses; it also stems from the difficulty of ruling them out as the culprit for various diseases. It is much harder to kill viruses than bacteria, so it has been impossible to eliminate viruses as suspects in certain disorders, even disorders such as multiple sclerosis that have been intensively studied. Further complicating the problem is the fact that humans are known to harbor many viruses that are in a quiescent state, even in the brain. For instance, most human brains contain latent cytomegalovirus and other herpes viruses. Added to the picture is the startling fact that some 8% of the human genome is made up of DNA sequences belonging to *human endogenous retroviruses*, known as HERVs. These sequences do not code for actual viruses; they are remnants of ancient retroviral infections that have persisted in our genome over the millennia. (An example of a retrovirus that is still active in humans is HIV.) The function of HERV sequences in our genome is still unknown and quite puzzling, but it is interesting that infections with other types of viruses can activate HERVs to make their corresponding RNAs. This shows that some HERV sequences, while normally latent, can be activated, although they do not typically make actual viruses. More familiar cases of latent viruses that can be activated are herpes viruses that mysteriously awake and cause cold sores or genital infections. It is also interesting, in light of our discussion in chapter 3 of the role of the placenta, that one of the HERVs codes for a protein that is predicted to mediate cell fusion during formation of the placental membrane that separates maternal and fetal tissues. Thus, at least one HERV could play a role in a key step in normal embryogenesis.

Although none of this information was available to the pioneers of schizophrenia research, they were clearly intrigued by what infections might do to human behavior. Emil Kraepelin speculated in his 1886 textbook that dementia praecox (early dementia) might be caused by an infection of another organ, with secondary effects on the brain. Eugen Bleuler later coined the term *schizophrenia*, recognizing that "dementia praecox" was inappropriate, given that schizophrenia was neither a dementia nor early in onset. Bleuler suggested that, "the connection of the disease [schizophrenia] to infectious processes equally needs further study . . . many writers assume that schizophrenia is caused by some physical weakness or possibly even by some infectious disease." As we saw in chapter 1, this is the line of thinking that led Wagner-Jauregg to test "pyrotherapy" in psychiatric disorders.

There is currently no strong evidence that infection in adults causes schizophrenia; however, it is clear that infections in children as well as adults can alter behavior. As discussed in chapter 2, this is seen most clearly in the sickness behavior that follows viral or bacterial infections of, for example, the lungs or urinary tract. We also learned that cytokines produced during infection, when injected into people, can induce major depression or even psychosis. Infections and immune activation have been implicated in childhood psychiatric disorders such as obsessive-compulsive disorder, Tourette's syndrome, attention deficit disorder, and an autoimmune disorder caused by streptococcal infection. Other examples of this phenomenon include the effects of some protozoan parasites; human behavior is strikingly altered by infection of *Plasmodium* (malaria) and *Trypanosoma* (sleeping sickness). Infection in pregnant women by the protozoan *Toxoplasma gondii* is implicated in the development of schizophrenia in the offspring—a fascinating connection that is discussed later in this chapter.

The most striking evidence that *T. gondii* can alter behavior in the adult comes from the work of Joanne Webster at Imperial College, London. The life story of this parasite is an example of the manipulation hypothesis, wherein a parasite alters its host's behavior for the parasite's benefit. The only known hosts in which *T. gondii* can reproduce sexually are felines. The parasite mates in the cat intestine, producing oocysts (thick-walled spores) that are then shed in the feces. These spores are very stable in the environment and are highly infectious when ingested. When the oocysts are eaten by an intermediate host such as a wild rodent or a human, they undergo asexual reproduction, resulting in infection of tissues such as the heart and brain. Lest one think that there is little exposure for humans, a study of meat samples in stores in England reported that 38% contained *T. gondii* oocysts! Contact with spores while cleaning cat litter boxes may also be a common source of infection. These cysts can remain latent and stable in tissues for the lifetime of the host. Transmission back to the definitive cat host then occurs when a cat eats the rodent, allowing the parasite to complete its life cycle in the cat intestine.

In most species studied, there appears to be little effect of the infection on the behavior of the intermediate host. A striking exception is found in rats and mice, which display a form of suicidal behavior in response to *T. gondii* infection. Normally, wild rats are innately neophobic, meaning that they avoid novel stimuli. This is the reason they are very difficult to trap or poison. Consistent with this trait, rats display a strong aversion to areas containing cat odors. In remarkable contrast, rats infected with *T. gondii* not only display a reduced aversion, but actually *prefer* to investigate areas containing cat odors. This behavior, of course, makes it easier for the cat to kill and eat the rodent that contains the *T. gondii* oocysts. Thus, the parasite has manipulated the host's behavior so as to be able to complete its life cycle by reproducing sexually in the cat's intestine.

An intriguing twist to this story is that the antipsychotic medication haloperidol, which is commonly used to treat schizophrenia, is the most potent inhibitor of *T. gondii* replication known. Moreover, treatment of *T. gondii*–infected rats with haloperidol restores their natural tendency to avoid areas containing cat odors. In light of the ability of cytokines to alter behavior, as discussed in chapter 2, it is also of interest that a latent *T. gondii* infection can permanently alter cytokine levels in the brain of the rodent host—perhaps due to a local immune response that keeps the *T. gondii* dormant. *T. gondii* is ubiquitous in humans; 70% or more display evidence of the parasite in their brains. Though it does not seem to cause major problems for the human host, the parasite can be reactivated by immunosuppression, for example by HIV infection or chemotherapy. Thus *T. gondii* could play a role in psychiatric problems found in AIDS patients.

There is also some recent evidence that children with high *T. gondii* levels display hyperactivity and low IQ. Given the widespread presence of the parasite, this is an observation that merits follow-up.

Maternal Infection and Schizophrenia

Although no substantive evidence connects infection in adults with schizophrenia, there is clear evidence linking infection in pregnant women with risk for schizophrenia in their offspring. Thus, it appears that this disorder can actually begin during embryogenesis. Because the initial, overt, psychotic symptoms are not manifested until early adulthood, it may seem surprising that schizophrenia is now generally considered to be a developmental disorder.

This view is based on several lines of evidence. First, retrospective studies of young children who are diagnosed with schizophrenia years later show that they tend to score poorly on cognitive tests. Second, these children can display slower motor development (of coordinated movements) and subtle signs of motor abnormalities, such as involuntary movements of the hand reminiscent of those made while playing the piano. The meaning of these motor observations is unclear, though they could be due to a disruption of development in the part of the brain that controls motor movements. Third, these children display an increased frequency of minor physical anomalies, particularly in the face and head. Such anomalies are known to be caused by problems during embryonic development, including maternal influenza infection. Fourth, some structural abnormalities in the brain that result from disruptions in embryonic development appear more frequently in schizophrenic subjects than in controls. Finally, MRI studies of the brains of young people deemed at high risk for developing the disorder show the presence of structural abnormalities before the onset of psychosis. (This population is thought to be at high risk because of schizophrenia in the family and the presence of abnormal symptoms in adolescence, such as hallucination-like voices.) Although none of these dysfunctions or abnormalities are specific to schizophrenia, nor can they be used as an early childhood test for schizophrenia, taken together the observations support the premise that schizophrenia is a disorder with origins in very early development.

What causes these early abnormalities and sets in motion the largely mysterious processes that eventuate in psychosis? One factor is genetics. As discussed in chapter 3, the concordance rate for schizophrenia in identical twins is 50%, a statistic that is usually taken to mean that genes have an important role in the disorder. In addition, several genes that are leading candidates for enhancing the risk for schizophrenia (e.g., *disrupted in schizophrenia 1*, or *DISC1*, and *neuregulin 1*) are known to play important roles in embryonic brain development. While mutations in most of the candidate genes confer very small effects on the risk for schizophrenia, DISC1 is an exception. The exceedingly rare families in which this gene is disabled display a very high frequency of mental illness, meaning that if a family member has the mutation, he or she is very likely to get such an illness. In this case, however, the mutation in DISC1 does not necessarily cause schizophrenia; it can also cause major depressive disorder or bipolar disorder. Why the same mutation causes these divergent disorders in various family members is not understood. It is possible that mutations in other genes interact with DISC1 to specify which disorder will develop. It is also possible that environmental factors interact with the DISC1 mutation to determine the type of disorder that will develop.

In fact, at least one environmental risk factor for schizophrenia is becoming well understood. In the 1950s and 1960s, Benjamin Pasamanick and E. Fuller Torrey each suggested that maternal infection should be investigated as a cause of schizophrenia. In the subsequent decades, many epidemiologic studies supported this notion, showing that being born during the winter or being born in an urban (versus a rural) area is associated with increased risk for schizophrenia. Although there are other possible explanations for these findings, both risk factors can be linked to an increased likelihood of infections by agents such as influenza and respiratory viruses. That is, pregnancy during winter or in a crowded urban environment increases the risk for infection in the mother as well as for schizophrenia in the offspring.

Such links received further support from the seminal 1988 paper by Sarnoff Mednick at the University of Southern California. Mednick's study of the 1957 influenza epidemic in Finland found that the offspring of women who were pregnant during this period had a significantly increased likelihood of becoming schizophrenic. Many subsequent studies of this and other flu epidemics in a variety of countries around the world further tested the association between influenza and schizophrenia in the offspring. Most papers confirmed this link; some did not. However, a major issue with most of these early studies was that infection was not confirmed in the pregnant women. That is, the fact that the epidemic passed through the city or country where they were living at the time did not mean that all of the pregnant women became infected. Moreover, the diagnosis of schizophrenia in the offspring was not confirmed by follow-up examinations.

This is why the work of Alan Brown at the Columbia College of Physicians and Surgeons is so important (see box 5.1). Brown, and Ezra Susser, and their colleagues overcame these obstacles by using blood samples taken from women during pregnancy. With this material they could determine which women had actually been infected, testing for the presence of antibodies against influenza virus and also for the presence of cytokines that go up during infection. Using these methods, they confirmed that maternal flu infection increases the risk for schizophrenia in the offspring three- to sevenfold. They also determined that the particular time window of vulnerability is in the first half of pregnancy. Infection during the second

Box 5.1
Alan Brown

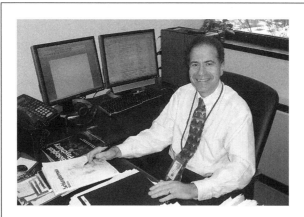

In a remarkable series of papers beginning in 2000, Alan Brown spearheaded the modern study of the connection between infection during pregnancy and

Box 5.1
(continued)

schizophrenia in the offspring. His findings indicate that many different pathogens can increase the risk for schizophrenia in the offspring, and he has proposed a series of public health preventative measures to decrease the prevalence of this tragic and costly mental illness. In addition, Brown's most recent findings suggest the possibility that there are different types of schizophrenia, depending on the cause. The ability to subdivide this heterogeneous illness based on objective, biological features will be a critical step forward in understanding its etiology and also for targeting individualized treatments, also known as personalized medicine.

As is true of many researchers, Brown's interest in science—especially astronomy—was apparent in early childhood, and his quantitative bent was evidenced by his memorization of the diameters of the planets. After college at Johns Hopkins University, he turned to medicine. Even as a first-year student at Jefferson Medical College, however, Brown realized that he wanted to do research, and he began to focus on the brain. He saw the increasing influence of basic neuroscience on psychiatry as an area of great potential for progress, and therefore did further training in psychiatry at the University of Pittsburgh, where excellent work in this area was taking place. While treating patients, Brown also managed to begin some laboratory work on the side.

The turning point in his career came in 1991 when he joined Ezra Susser at the New York Psychiatric Institute, which is affiliated with the Columbia College of Physicians and Surgeons. Susser's work on the epidemiology of the Dutch Hunger Winter was under way at that time, and Sarnoff Mednick, working at the University of Southern California, had recently published his important early study suggesting a link between influenza infection in pregnant women and schizophrenia in the offspring. With early funding from the National Alliance for Research on Schizophrenia and Depression, and a fellowship from the National Institutes of Health, Brown utilized the Child Health and Development Study as the basis for the prospective investigation of the maternal infection risk factor. This involved access to the invaluable resource of archived serum samples taken from women at each trimester of pregnancy. The investigators could therefore confirm when infections had taken place, and they could then predict the critical window of vulnerability of the fetus to the dangers of infection in the mother.

Brown was promoted to the faculty at Columbia in 1994 and has remained there ever since. His major research interest remains in the area of developmental neurobiology. Most recently, his work has included the study of environmental risk factors for autism. (Photo by Paul Patterson) half was found to convey no increased risk for schizophrenia in the off-spring. (Many other studies have shown, however, that maternal infection late in pregnancy does carry risk for other types of diseases, such as cystic fibrosis.)

Another important finding has come out of the work by Brown and colleagues. They have recently examined the schizophrenia subjects in their cohort, both those who were born to mothers who were infected during pregnancy and those born to mothers who did not experience such infections. They examined the subjects with a variety of cognitive tests and also with MRI. The results showed that the schizophrenic subjects who were born to mothers who had been infected performed differently on several cognitive tests than the schizophrenic subjects who were born to mothers without infections. In addition, those born to infected mothers also more frequently displayed a structural abnormality in the brain that earlier had been shown to occur in schizophrenia—notably, a structural abnormality that is known to be caused by problems in embryonic development. These differences between the schizophrenic subjects born to infected and noninfected mothers suggest the possibility that different causes of schizophrenia can lead to diverse phenotypes (differing neuropathology and behavioral deficits). It is well known that there is considerable heterogeneity in the symptoms of schizophrenia, and it would be a great step forward to begin to explain how this variety arises, so as to be able separate out different types of schizophrenia, a process that could eventually lead to different treatment protocols.

Although influenza infection is the most widely studied maternal risk factor (because of the frequency of infection and the periodicity of epidemics), it is not the only maternal infection associated with risk for schizophrenia in the offspring. Another early study by Brown documented maternal infection by the rubella (German measles) virus and found a significant increase in schizophrenia in those offspring, particularly if the infection occurred during early pregnancy. Maternal infection with *T. gondii* (the parasite in cat litter boxes) is also linked to schizophrenia in the offspring. This was shown by tests of archived blood samples, taken during pregnancy or from newborns, for elevated levels of antibodies against the parasite, which is a sign of a recent, active infection. There is also evidence that genital infection by herpes virus during pregnancy increases the risk for schizophrenia in the offspring. Maternal bacterial infection is yet another infection risk for the disorder. Thus, the risk of maternal infection is not confined to influenza or even to viruses. Rather, it is maternal infection itself that is the key. As discussed in the next chapter, work with animal models suggests that it is the mother's inflammatory response to infection that is critical for altering fetal brain development.

As discussed in more detail in chapter 9, these various infections during pregnancy are now estimated to account for over a third of all schizophrenia cases, so this is a serious public health concern. Chapter 9 also takes up the question of how to prevent such infections.

Maternal Infection and Autism

The man who named schizophrenia, Eugen Bleuler, also coined the term *autismus* (from the Greek: *autos*, self) in 1910 as he was defining the symptoms of schizophrenia. Leo Kanner of the Johns Hopkins Hospital first used the term *autism* in its modern sense in English when he introduced the label *early infantile autism* in a 1943 report of 11 children with striking behavioral similarities. Kanner originally classified autism as a subtype of schizophrenia. This had largely to do with the negative symptoms of the latter disorder—lack of adequate social interaction, poverty of speech—and the apparent focus inward, on oneself. Of course, the two disorders can be distinguished by other symptoms, such as delusions and hallucinations in schizophrenia versus severely restricted interests, highly repetitive behaviors, and the absence of language development (or early regression of language) in autism. The age of onset of easily observable symptoms is very different as well, typically being around 3 years for autism and late or post-adolescence for schizophrenia, although a small subset of schizophrenia patients display psychosis in childhood. Both disorders are highly heterogeneous, which is reflected in the term used to label the broader group of symptoms in autism, *autism spectrum disorders* (ASD). Despite the differences in behavioral symptoms, autism and schizophrenia share a number of features of importance for our purposes here. One such feature is the involvement of immune abnormalities, as discussed in chapter 7. Another is the maternal infection risk factor.

Although the number of large epidemiologic studies looking for autism risk factors lags far behind that for schizophrenia, there is evidence for the involvement of maternal infection in the former disorder. Initial support for this notion came from research on the 1964 rubella pandemic, in which Stella Chase at the New York University Medical Center reported that the incidence of autistic features (lack of communication, stereotyped and asocial behaviors) was increased more than 200-fold in the offspring of infected mothers. Of course, due to the subsequent routine use of childhood rubella vaccination, dangerous rubella infections in pregnant women are now rare and not a cause of autism. However, these epidemics did provide proof of the principle that maternal infection can cause large increases in the incidence of autistic features in the offspring. We also have evidence that the window of vulnerability for autism is different from that in schizophrenia. The autism outcome is more frequent if infection (or ingestion of the teratogen thalidomide) occurs early in the first trimester, whereas a schizophrenia outcome is more frequent following infection late in the first trimester or early in the second trimester. It should not be at all surprising, of course, that infections at different stages of fetal brain development would lead to different postnatal behavioral outcomes. And in fact, animal studies of the maternal infection risk factor confirm that the timing of infection is critical for the eventual behavioral symptoms (see chapter 6).

In addition to rubella, case studies (small studies of just one or a few patients) have linked autism to several other maternal viral infections, including varicella, rubeola, and cytomegalovirus. Bacterial and protozoan infections have also been associated with autism. The most comprehensive study to date, however, is one that surveyed the medical records of all children born in Denmark between 1980 and 2005, including more than 10,000 children diagnosed with ASD. The analysis by Hjördis Atladóttir and colleagues at the University of Aarhus in Denmark revealed a significant association of autism with first-trimester maternal *viral* infection and with second-trimester maternal *bacterial* infection. This study is important not only because of the huge size of the cohort, but also because it employed modern diagnostic criteria to characterize the symptoms. The apparent discrepancy between the timing of vulnerability between viral and bacterial infection is provocative. Both types of infection evoke an immune response in the mother, but the response is slightly different in its components. Perhaps study of these details could shed light on which key molecules are important in predisposing a child to autism? This is an area where the use of animal models, discussed in the next chapter, could be very helpful.

If maternal infection is an important risk factor, why don't all children born to mothers who experience an infection during pregnancy go on to develop autism or schizophrenia? In fact, except for the case of rubella, only a small proportion of such offspring develop these disorders. There are two obvious explanations, and both are very likely to have merit. First, the degree of the infection and/or the degree of the mother's inflammatory response is important. A flu infection can lead to loss of a day's work or it can lead to a week or more of bed rest, or even hospitalization. The same is true for urinary tract infections, for instance. Rubella, on the other hand, is a uniformly severe infection, and the offspring display a range of very serious problems including physical abnormalities as well as deafness and mental retardation. Thus, it is not surprising that the frequency of autistic symptoms in these children is reported to be far higher than in the off-spring of mothers with other types of infection.

The second key factor in the outcome of maternal infection is likely to be genetics. Both autism and schizophrenia are known to have a strong genetic component, although it has been extremely difficult to isolate the key genes that influence risk. Nonetheless, several recent studies that scanned the entire human genome for variants of genes that may be associated with schizophrenia did localize one area of interest. This turned out to be in a region coding for the major compatibility complex, or MHC (as well as several other genes). Recall from chapter 2 that MHC proteins are involved in the immune response to infection. If a cell is infected with a virus, and its MHC protein displays a peptide from that virus on the cell surface, the cell will be killed. This effectively stops that cell from being a productive host for viral replication. One implication of the association between MHC and schizophrenia risk is that genes in this part of the chromosome could possibly play a role in the response to maternal infection and thereby influence the risk of schizophrenia.

Several single-gene mutations convey increased risk for the development of autistic symptoms. These mutations do not necessarily cause classical autism; rather, they may cause autistic symptoms coupled with a variety of other pathologies not found in autism. An example of this type of condition is the rare disorder *tuberous sclerosis* (TSC; from the Latin: *tuber*, swelling; and Greek: *skleros*, hard), a genetic disease in which mutations in one of two TSC genes cause multiple, benign tumors to grow in various tissues including the brain. These mutations in TSC can be effectively created in mice, providing a mouse disease model that displays features of the human disorder. Alcino Silva and colleagues at the University of California at Los Angeles used this mouse model to look for interactions between a TSC mutation and the maternal infection risk factor. In this experiment, pregnant mice were given injections of either saline (as a control) or an agent that evokes an inflammatory response much like that seen when the mice are given a respiratory infection with the flu virus. The adult offspring are then tested for behaviors relevant for autism. This study is discussed in more detail in the following chapter; the key point here is that the offspring carrying the mutant TSC gene display autistic-like behavior, but only if they were born to mothers that were immune activated during pregnancy. That is, abnormal behavior was not seen in TSC-mutant offspring born to mothers that were injected with saline during pregnancy. The abnormal behavior was also not seen in normal mice (not carrying the TSC mutation) born to mothers that were immune activated during pregnancy. Thus, it takes a combination of both maternal immune activation and the TSC mutation to get the effect on behavior in these mice. This could be due to an effect of the TSC mutation on the function of the immune system, making it more susceptible or reactive to the maternal immune activation.

Another such interaction between genetic background and maternal infection involves urinary tract infections and schizophrenia. In a recent investigation of Finnish medical records, Mary Clarke and Mary Cannon at the Royal College of Surgeons in Ireland found that maternal urinary tract infection nearly doubles the risk of schizophrenia in people with a family history of psychosis compared to people with a family history but no such infection. Thus, the combination of presumed genetic susceptibility coupled with maternal infection significantly increases risk.

How does infection during pregnancy alter fetal brain development such that the offspring are at risk for mental illness? That question is considered in the next chapter.

6   Animal Models of Autism, Schizophrenia, and Depression?

There is a wonderful kind of excitement in modern neuroscience, a romantic, moonwalk sense of exploring and setting out for new frontiers. The science is elegant, the scientists dismayingly young, and the pace of discovery absolutely staggering. . . . It would take a mind that is on empty, or a heart made of stone, to be unmoved by their collective ventures and enthusiasms.

—K. R. Jamison, *An Unquiet Mind*

Schizophrenic Mice?

The title of this chapter is a bit of a straw man. It is not possible to create mouse models of these brain disorders that *completely* mimic those in humans, any more than it is possible to discuss symptoms with the animal "patient" (see figure 6.1). This is not because mice and monkeys, for instance, fail to share brain structure and functions with humans—they do. Nor is it because such animals are not capable of learning—they are. It is because mice, for example, have different strengths and weaknesses than humans. Humans have a relatively underdeveloped olfactory system and depend largely on the visual system; mice have a relatively underdeveloped visual system and rely very heavily on their olfactory sense. Mice also utilize their whiskers for sensing the world around them, especially in the dark, whereas most humans shave off their whiskers or don't have any facial hair to begin with! Correspondingly, the regions of the brain that subserve these senses in the mouse are more or less strongly represented than in the human, and so it is difficult to transfer the various tests used to measure cognitive abilities in humans directly to mice. Social memory, for example, may be primarily visual in humans but primarily olfactory in mice. Such differences necessitate rethinking how to make the tests used in the two species directly comparable.

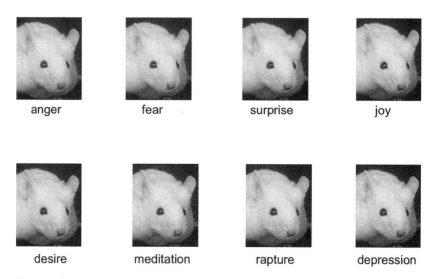

| anger | fear | surprise | joy |

| desire | meditation | rapture | depression |

Figure 6.1
The ease with which one can infer what a mouse is thinking is apparent from these pictures. (From P. H. Patterson)

Then there is the issue of language and communication. A primary means of measuring cognitive abilities in humans is through language-based tests. And, although scientists are still trying to decipher the meaning of all the various calls emitted by nonhuman primates and dolphins, among other animals, it seems unlikely that these calls carry the rich complexity of the verbal communications that humans know as language. Nonhuman primates, for example, can make calls that are used for warning the group of the presence of particular types of predators; however, it seems doubtful that they carry on discussions of abstract topics such as the meaning of life and the creation of the universe. When considering mental illnesses such as autism, major depressive disorder, and schizophrenia, the lack of language in laboratory animals presents a major stumbling block in constructing experimental animal models. This is not to say, as some have, that schizophrenia and autism are uniquely human disorders. How can we know that they are uniquely human? In fact, the evidence suggests that animals such as mice and monkeys can indeed experience some of the features of psychiatric disorders. Much of the research described in this chapter concerns how to assess whether an animal is displaying such symptoms.

In spite of the hurdles, truly remarkable progress has been made in developing and utilizing mouse models of a variety of human brain diseases, such as Alzheimer's and Huntington's diseases. This is because genetic models can be made of these disorders. Huntington's disease is a true genetic disease, meaning that if you inherit a particular mutation in the gene called *huntingtin*, you get the disease. Because genetic manipulations can be made very efficiently in mice (not the case in monkeys), it is possible to introduce this human mutation into mice and then study their behavior and neuropathology. The latter term refers to the signs of cell death and disruption of neuron structure and brain circuits that can be visualized under the microscope. Indeed, when mutant huntingtin is introduced into the genome of a particular strain of mice (producing "transgenic mice"), they develop movement abnormalities reminiscent of those in the human disease, such as loss of balance and coordination and the ability to climb easily. They also exhibit several classic signs of neuropathology that are found in Huntington's. These mice are extremely valuable, as they faithfully pass the mutant human gene on to their progeny, making it possible to send a reproducible mouse model around the world so that various laboratories, with different types of expertise, can study them.

The case of Alzheimer's disease mouse models is somewhat different, because Alzheimer's is not usually a true genetic disease, and its causes are not at all well understood. Nonetheless, a small percentage of Alzheimer's cases are due to mutations, and when those mutations are introduced into mice, the transgenic mice develop signs of the disease. These signs include a deficit in the ability to learn and remember, as well as the classic signs of Alzheimer's neuropathology, senile plaques, and tangles. (Plaques are large deposits of proteins that can be stained with certain dyes. Tangles are twisted clumps of neuronal extensions.) On the other hand, these mice do not display all of the signs of the human disorder. For instance, they do not show the specific loss of certain types of neurons that occurs in human Alzheimer's disease. The important lesson here is, however, that it is possible to model particular *features* of human brain diseases in mice. Moreover, this process is now straightforward for genetic diseases, where transgenic lines of mice can be produced. Such models have proven extremely useful in the investigation of what goes wrong in the circuits of the brain in those disorders, and of what types of treatments can alleviate the symptoms. Experiments of the latter type are leading to human clinical trials of treatments that were first discovered and tested in mice (see chapter 9). Work with animals has also led to the discovery of a great many cellular and molecular pathways that underlie the neuropathology and abnormal behaviors in these diseases, in turn enabling a greater understanding of how the *healthy* brain works. In sum, these mouse models, while imperfect, are enormously useful.

Therefore, when considering mental illness the question becomes, can we model *features* of these disorders in animals? Can we see behavioral symptoms or neuropathology in mice or nonhuman primates that resemble those in human autism, schizophrenia, or major depressive disorder? The broader, if imprecise, question that is often asked is, how does one tell if a mouse is schizophrenic?

Despite the daunting complexity and considerable heterogeneity in schizophrenia, autism, and depression, it is possible to make a list of the major hallmarks of each disorder, and then see if one can realistically test for those features in animals. For schizophrenia, the negative symptoms (loss of normal functions) include disorganized thinking (deficits in executive function, described below) and deficits in learning and memory, in displays of emotion, in verbal communication, and in social interaction. The positive symptoms (functions that appear) include hallucinations and delusions. One of the most often reproduced neuropathologic findings in schizophrenia is an expansion of the ventricles, the fluid-filled cavities in the center of the brain. The cerebral cortex is also found to be deficient in *parvalbumin*, a protein that is thought to be important in the electrical rhythms that underlie cognitive function. Turning to animal models, it is quite straightforward to stain thinly cut sections of the brains of mice, for instance, to detect neurons that produce parvalbumin. It is also possible to measure the size of the ventricles in these brains, as well as to investigate other types of neuropathology seen in human schizophrenia. Although none of these neuropathologies is specific to schizophrenia, finding them in a mouse model would support the hypothesis that the model is showing features of schizophrenia.

It is also possible to adapt human behavioral tests for use with rodents. For instance, there are many different ways of testing for deficits in learning and memory in mice. Some of the tasks involve remembering a particular odor or having met a particular mouse before, or remembering where to look for a hidden food pellet. Since mice do not like to swim, they can also be tested for the ability to remember where to find a platform hidden just under the surface of a large pool of water in which they are swimming; finding the platform enables them to stand up out of the water. Mice use spatial cues in the room, such as pictures on the walls, to orient themselves in the pool. If these cues are moved after the mouse learns where the platform is located (a nasty trick), the mouse goes to the wrong location in the pool in search of the platform. Such tests, and other, more sophisticated ones involving touching the nose to different icons on a small computer screen in order to receive a food or juice reward, can be used to test for memory deficits that are potentially similar to those in schizophrenia.

It is also possible to test for deficits in executive function, which can be defined as the ability to coordinate responses in accordance with changing external demands or rules. One assay for this type of brain function in humans is the Wisconsin Card Sorting Test. In this paradigm, a person is rewarded for discovering and following an unspoken rule for sorting cards, say by color. Without telling the subject, the tester then changes the rule to now reward by sorting by number. The time it takes for the subject to recognize this and adapt to the new rule is measured. This assessment of "frontal lobe" brain function tests abilities such as strategic planning, organized searching, utilizing environmental feedback to shift a cognitive framework, directing behavior toward achieving a goal, and modulating impulsive responses. The test can be effectively administered to children as well as the elderly. Schizophrenic subjects have great difficulty in dynamically updating and integrating new information in this test. Similarly, mice can be tested for their ability to adapt to reversal of the rules for obtaining rewards. They may be rewarded with a food pellet for looking in a particular location or for turning right at a choice point. When the reward is then reset to a new location or at the left turn for the food, the time taken to learn the new rule is measured.

Social interaction can also be measured in mice. In one test, the subject is placed in the central chamber of a three-chamber box whose walls are transparent. There are open passages to the other two chambers, of which one is empty and the other contains an unfamiliar mouse in a wire cage. A typical mouse will spend more time investigating the new mouse than investigating the empty chamber. This is taken to be a preference for social interaction or investigation. Investigation of a novel, inanimate object in one side chamber versus investigation of a novel mouse in the other side chamber is another version of a social test.

Schizophrenia patients also tend to exhibit difficulties with attention, and often can be easily distracted. One test for this type of problem is termed *prepulse inhibition*. In humans and in mice this can be assessed by measuring the amount of startle to a loud sound (the animal jumps a bit) or to a puff of air to the eye (the human flinches). If this startle stimulus is preceded by a much softer sound or puff of air, the amount of startle is normally diminished, as if the smaller stimulus "prepared" the subject for being startled. Hence the name, prepulse inhibition of the acoustic (or somatosensory) startle. Schizophrenic subjects have deficits in prepulse inhibition. That is, their level of startle is not diminished by the prestimulus.

As is the case for the neuropathology, deficits in any of these behavioral tests are not specific to schizophrenia; such deficits in individual tests can also be found in disorders such as autism or attention deficit hyperactivity disorder, for instance. Nonetheless, the presence of such deficits in the animal would reinforce the hypothesis that the mouse model is exhibiting features of schizophrenia. Researchers can also ask if the mouse behavior in question appears in early adulthood, as is the case in schizophrenia, and whether the behavioral deficit responds to known antipsychotic drugs. Experimenters can also use these behavioral tests to examine the efficacy of potential, new antipsychotic (in the case of schizophrenia) drugs. However, there is always guesswork involved in pinpointing the aspect of schizophrenia symptoms to which an animal behavior test is directly relevant.

Are there any symptoms that are specific to schizophrenia, and therefore could be used definitively to identify a feature in an animal model as being linked to this disorder in particular? The more specific symptoms of schizophrenia are the positive ones: hallucinations and delusions. There are, however, other disorders that are possibly related to schizophrenia and that also occasionally exhibit hallucinations, such as bipolar disorder. Nonetheless, it would be of great interest to be able to study hallucinations in animals such as mice. But if a mouse cannot tell us what it is thinking, how would we know whether it is hallucinating? A useful, practical definition of a hallucination is neuronal activity in the sensory cerebral cortex (visual or auditory systems) in the absence of sensory input (e.g., with the subject placed in a dark and silent room). In addition, such brain activity should resemble that which is seen when an animal subject is given a known hallucinogen such as LSD. But how do we determine where and when brain activity is increased? Fortunately, there are a variety of ways of assessing neural activity in the brains of animals. Functional MRI is one method commonly used in humans, and it can also be used in monkeys. It is difficult to use with conscious mice, however, because they struggle when restrained in a setting like an MRI scanner. Their movements prevent accurate images from being collected. Our laboratory and others are working on ways to circumvent these problems.

Another method for monitoring brain activity is to implant an array containing multiple microelectrodes into the brain. This is done in humans for the purpose of localizing the source of epileptic seizures, for instance. Such array implants have uncovered a number of interesting findings in humans, such as individual neurons that fire electrical impulses only when the patient is shown various pictures of Jennifer Aniston, for instance. Such neurons do not fire in response to other actresses or other people. Most compelling is the finding that the same neurons also fire in response to the subject being shown the name "Jennifer Aniston." Other individual neurons in this part of the brain can fire specifically in response to pictures of other famous people that are familiar to the person being tested. While we are all aware of our ability to recognize specific people, it is nonetheless startling to discover that this capacity can be exhibited in individual neurons. When our gray matter shrinks in schizophrenia, or in normal aging, is it any surprise that there are decrements in memory?

Whether mouse neurons would respond to pictures of Jennifer Aniston after having seen her movies is an open question. However, it has been shown in monkeys that individual neurons in the so-called face areas of the brain can respond to specific monkey faces, some responding selectively to familiar faces, some to unfamiliar faces. The search for possible parallels with human face recognition is under way.

An entirely different technique for visualizing neural activity in the brain involves the analysis of gene expression. Certain genes are turned on to make RNA and protein immediately after the neuron is stimulated and starts firing. Such genes are termed *immediate early genes* (IEGs) because of this very fast response. The activity of the IEGs can be monitored globally in the brain when the animal is sacrificed and its brain sliced into thin sections. These sections are then stained for the RNA or protein products of the IEGs. Using this technique as a surrogate measure of neuronal activity, our laboratory and others have found that injection of a hallucinogen into mice induces IEG activation specifically in the sensory cortex, in the absence of visual or auditory stimulation. Thus, it may be possible to make some progress toward evaluating even the seemingly most elusive schizophrenia symptoms in mice.

What about modeling features of autism in mice? As with schizophrenia, the task seems insurmountable at first. The primary symptoms are lack (or regressive loss) of language, deficits in social interaction, stereotyped, repetitive behaviors, and narrow interests coupled with a desire for sameness. The disorder can also include seizures, enhanced anxiety under mildly stressful conditions, disturbed sleep patterns, gastrointestinal (GI) disturbances, altered pain sensitivity, and deficits in prepulse inhibition. Neuropathologies that are frequently seen in autism include a Purkinje cell deficit that is restricted to a particular region of the cerebellum, as well as characteristic neurochemical changes (notably abnormalities in serotonin, a chemical neurotransmitter used in communication between neurons in certain parts of the brain and also found in the GI tract and in platelets in the blood). As with schizophrenia, there is a great deal of heterogeneity in the range of symptoms found in individuals diagnosed with autism, and even more diversity if one includes autism spectrum disorders (ASD). Moreover, some of these symptoms overlap with schizophrenia, such as enhanced anxiety, deficits in social interaction, and altered sensory functions and prepulse inhibition. As discussed previously, these latter symptoms have been successfully modeled in mice.

What about the other symptoms in autism; can they be modeled in mice? Stereotyped, repetitive behaviors can certainly be assessed in mice. One example of this is excessive repetitive grooming. Another test that has been used is a marble-burying task. When a normal mouse is placed in a cage with many glass marbles sitting on top of the wood-chip bedding, it will bury some of them. In contrast, in a model of autistic features (induced by maternal infection; described below), the mouse buries all of the marbles quickly. Some investigators liken this behavior to obsessive-compulsive disorder.

Desire for sameness can also be described as neophobia, or fear of the new. This has been assayed in mice by testing the time spent investigating a novel object. Typical mice are very curious about novel objects, while, as we shall see, some mouse models of autism do not display this trait. Another feature often seen in autism is seizures, and these can be monitored effectively in mice, as can seizure threshold—the amount of an injected convulsive chemical that is needed to induce a seizure. For the characteristic neuropathology in autism involving a deficit in the very large neurons in the cerebellum, the Purkinje cells, these cells can be counted in tissue slices and the findings directly compared with the human neuropathology.

The major stumbling block in thinking about animal models in the context of autism is the perplexing and frustrating lack of language in many cases of autism. Notwithstanding the Gary Larsen cartoon in which two cows are seen standing on their hind legs, one saying, "Better get down on all fours, here comes a car," there are no reports of mice being overheard using words to converse in their cages late at night when they are most active. On the other hand, mice do emit squeaks when they are mishandled or in pain, but these are not of interest in the present context. More intriguing are the vocalizations that mice and rats emit in the ultrasonic frequency range. This is the range of frequencies that bats use as sonar to detect their insect prey. That is why "bat detector" equipment is used to monitor mouse ultrasonic vocalizations (USVs). Such recordings have highlighted two conditions in which mice vocalize particularly often. In one case, young mouse pups vocalize actively when they are removed from their nest. This important signal helps the mother to find the missing pup, exemplifying mother-infant social communication. In adult mice, males vocalize frequently when they meet a female or are given the scent of a female, as in a urine sample. It is not yet clear whether such calls are meant to communicate with the female or are just cries of excitement.

Some researchers are exploring the information that may be contained in such USVs. In our own laboratory, Natalia Malkova, Collin Yu, and others are analyzing the calls by studying the distribution of their frequencies. The analogy is with birdsong. In most songbird species, only the males sing and the young son learns its song from its father. These songs are in the audible human range of frequencies, and analysis of the distribution of the frequencies has shown that the young birds go through an initial "babbling" phase and then gradually refine their song to match that of their fathers. This song development requires that the young bird hear its own vocalizations, so that it can mimic the memory of the song it heard from its father (or from a recording of that song played back by an experimenter). They key point of interest in terms of mice is that bird songs can be analyzed by the distribution of the frequencies of the calls. Individual syllables and phrases can be characterized, and these are put together in a highly reproducible order in the song, which is distinct for each songbird species (figure 6.2). When the same type of analysis was applied to the USVs of adult male mice, Tim Holy of the Washington University of St. Louis Medical School reported that each individual male had his own distinctive "song" of syllables and phrases, which remains stable over time. This intriguing claim needs to be further investigated.

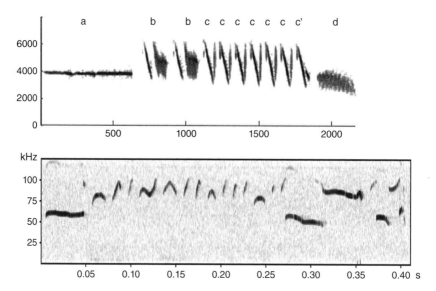

Figure 6.2
Upper panel: A sound spectrogram analysis of a typical song of a white-crowned sparrow is shown (frequency on the vertical axis versus time in milliseconds on the horizontal axis). The smallest elements, the notes, are combined to form syllables (lowercase letters), and these are repeated to form phrases. White-crowned sparrow songs typically begin with (a) a long whistle followed by (b, c) trills and (d) buzzes. (From Doupe and Kuhl, 1999.) Lower panel: A spectrogram of a series of ultrasonic vocalizations from a male mouse (frequency versus time in seconds). Although the individual syllables are not reproduced as precisely as in the bird, it is possible to recognize and quantify them. (From Collin Yu and Natalia Malkova)

What could be the biological function of such mouse songs? In the case of the songbirds, it is thought that there are species-specific songs but not songs specific to individual birds (except in unusual cases such as parrots). Such songs are known to be important for defense of territory and for courting females. If it is true that mice produce reproducible songs that differ among individuals, they could potentially be used for recognition and communication. These songs would not be learned from the male offspring's fathers because, in most cases, the father has been removed from the cage of the pregnant female; even if he were there, presumably he would be "teaching" his whole litter of pups the same song. Thus, individual songs among male mice would indicate that the source of the mouse "songs" is different from that of birdsong.

Another extremely intriguing finding in the area of animal communication involves the discovery of a gene that is required for verbal communication in humans. The KE family in England was found to have developmental verbal dyspraxia, a speech and language disorder that compromises the fluent production of words and the correct use and comprehension of grammar. The gene whose mutation causes the disorder in this family is called *FOXP2*. The FOXP2 gene is important for the present discussion because its DNA sequence is strongly conserved from reptiles to humans, including birds and mice. This strict conservation suggests that it has maintained its function(s) during evolution. The expression, and hence function, of FOXP2 is increased in the songbird brain during the time of vocal learning. Moreover, when the gene's expression is experimentally knocked down during this period, the mature bird from that experiment displays an incomplete and inaccurate imitation of its tutor song. This shows that FOXP2 is important in learning or maintaining the song. Among mammalian species, the sequence of the FOXP2 gene and protein is among the most highly conserved, indicating it has a fundamental role in these animals as well. Since mice and humans diverged during evolution 70 million years ago, there have been only three small changes in the FOXP2 sequence.

Thus, it was of interest to replace the mouse FOXP2 with the human version of the gene. Would the mice now talk? If so, autism symptoms would be much easier to study in mice! Of course, it would also raise a few very uncomfortable ethical issues for research on these mice. For better or worse, Svante Paabo and his team in Germany found that the mice expressing the human FOXP2 gene did not talk. However, when the pups were removed from their mother, their USVs did display an altered structure in comparison to normal mice. Since the part of the mouse brain that drives vocalizations differs somewhat from that in the human, and the structure and mechanics of the mouth and throat differ between the two species, it is absurd to imagine that changing one gene in the brain could have a genuine humanizing effect on mouse vocalizations. Nonetheless, changing the FOXP2 gene sequence very slightly did have a subtle effect on the USVs of the mice.

Obviously, much fascinating work remains to be done in the area of animal vocalizations. But already, an amazing variety of experiments are being done in mice that allow us to compare some of the symptoms in autism and schizophrenia to analogous behaviors in mice.

Mouse Models of Features of Major Depressive Disorder

What about tests in rodents that are meant to mimic behavioral symptoms of major depressive disorder? One that has been mentioned previously is the forced swim test. In this type of study, the mouse or rat is placed in a beaker of water from which it cannot escape. In this test of "behavioral despair," the time it takes for the animal to become immobile (or the time spent being immobile) is measured. The major evidence that this is relevant for depression is that a wide variety of clinically effective antidepressant medications are able to reduce the immobility time in this test—the animal does not give up as easily.

Another feature of depression that is modeled in rodents is termed *anhedonia* (from the Greek: *an*, without; *hedone*, pleasure). This core symptom of the human disorder is described as a "markedly diminished interest or pleasure in nearly all activities most of the day, nearly every day." One way of measuring anhedonia in rodents is to offer them a choice between water and a sucrose solution. While normal mice prefer the sweet drink, this preference is strikingly diminished if the animal has undergone chronic stress. This change is interpreted as a reduction in the "reward" experienced by the animal in a formerly pleasurable activity. This intuitively seems analogous to the situation in major depressive disorder, where the patient has lost interest in formerly pleasurable activities. And in fact, in stressed animals the preference for sucrose can be reestablished by chronic treatment with antidepressant medications that are similarly effective in humans.

Repeated stressful events can predispose people to depression. As was discussed in chapter 2, chronic stress can reset the level of receptors for the hormone cortisol in the brain by activating the hypothalamic-pituitary-adrenal (HPA) axis. Recall that the HPA axis is at the crossroads between the brain and peripheral organs. Chronic activation of the HPA axis raises cortisol and lowers receptors for this hormone in the hippocampus. Chronic stress can also change the rate of addition of new neurons to the hippocampus, which is normally ongoing in the adult brain. It is thought that the addition of new neurons is important for learning and possibly other cognitive functions. Several different animal models have been developed that show how stress can alter the HPA axis, with subsequent effects on behavior and on the production of new neurons.

For instance, *chronic administration of a cortisol-like corticosteroid* raises the hormone in mice to a higher, stable level, as is seen in some patients with depression. This results in increased symptoms of anxiety as well as immobility in the forced swim test. These mice also exhibit decreased grooming behavior, a type of personal neglect that is found in a subset of depressed patients. In addition, these mice display an altered circadian rhythm, which is common in human depression. The normal addition of new neurons in the adult hippocampus is markedly slowed as well. Many of these symptoms can be reversed in this mouse model by chronic, but not acute, treatment with antidepressant medications. The latter point is of interest because in treatment of human major depression, these medications must be taken for more than a week before they begin to alleviate symptoms. This is surprising because the SSRI (selective serotonin reuptake inhibitor) medications block uptake of serotonin almost immediately after administration. The reason for the delay in symptom relief is not yet understood, but animal models are being used to test various theories. One idea is that blocking the uptake results in changes in gene expression—alterations in certain RNAs and then in the corresponding proteins produced in the brain. It is these changes in protein levels that may then affect the behavioral symptoms of depression. Another effect of SSRI treatment in rodents is to increase the number of new neurons produced in the hippocampus. Similarly in humans, an increase in neural precursor cells has been seen. This is a critical line of experimental investigation because once the underlying molecular basis for the action of these medications is clarified, more effective and selective drugs may be developed, with fewer side effects. In addition, overcoming the delay in relieving symptoms is of particular importance for patients experiencing suicidal thoughts. Moreover, the current medications are ineffective in some 30% of severely depressed patients. Thus, there is a genuine need for more efficacious medications.

A related rodent model that also manipulates the HPA axis involves exposure to *unpredictable chronic mild stress*. Such stressors, presented in random order over days or weeks, include exposure to cold temperatures or bright lights, swimming in a pool, or having the cage placed on a slowly rotating table. These protocols result in elevated levels of a cortisol-like hormone and lowered levels of its receptor in the hippocampus. One of consequences is an anhedonic state, which can be reversed by chronic treatment with antidepressant medications. Depressive-like behavior is also observed in the forced swim test.

Another animal model is based on *adverse early life* experiences, which can predispose humans to depression in adulthood. As discussed in chapter 4, one way of modeling this effect in rodents involves dysfunctional parenting. For instance, the offspring of mothers who are poor at licking and grooming their pups are compared with the offspring of mothers who spend more time doing so. Poor maternal care results in adult offspring that display hyperresponsiveness to stress due to alterations in the HPA axis and the cortisol receptors in the hippocampus. As adults, these female offspring will also go on to display less nurturing behavior with their young.

Another way to create adverse early life experience is to separate the pups from the mother for a certain period of time each day. This disruption in maternal care can result in depression-like behavior in the offspring. There are also alterations in the HPA axis, the level of cortisol receptors, and the responses to stress in the adult offspring. Moreover, production of new neurons in the hippocampus is lower in the adult offspring, and more frequent cell death has been observed as well. A third animal model of early life stress involves stressing the pregnant rodent. The offspring of these mothers also display many of the same features that are seen in the other models. Recall that severe stress during human pregnancy has been found to increase the risk for schizophrenia in the offspring.

In addition to these models based on manipulation of the environment, many genetic models are being developed. More than 80 different strains of genetically modified mice have been found to display anxiety- and/or depression-like behaviors. These animals are extremely valuable resources with which to study the molecular basis of such behaviors and to test novel antidepressant drugs. A number of the genetic modifications in these mice are based on the roles that particular genes and proteins are known to play in human depression. The most obvious target is the gene that codes for the protein that removes serotonin from the synaptic connection between two neurons. This is the *serotonin transporter*. When serotonin is removed from the synapse connecting two neurons, its action on its receptor protein is terminated. Thus, when SSRI medications that block the transporter are given for depression, serotonin lasts longer in the synapse and is likely to have more effect on its receptor. Since these medications can be effective in major depressive disorder, it suggests that a critical issue in this disorder is serotonin action at the synapse (or within neurons; blocking uptake also affects the level of serotonin inside neurons). In fact, as discussed in chapter 2, people who have a particular genetic variant of the serotonin transporter (the short form) are more likely to respond to repeated stressful events by becoming very depressed and even suicidal than are people who have another variant of this transporter (the long form). In addition, the variants in the serotonin transporter gene are associated with the therapeutic responses to SSRI treatment as well as the side effects of the medications. Thus, the type of serotonin receptor a person has can influence a number of characteristics that are important in depression.

Therefore, one of the first genetic manipulations in mice relevant for depression was to knock out (inactivate) the serotonin transporter gene. This would be expected to have effects similar to those seen in people with the short form of the serotonin transporter gene, which is less effective at taking up serotonin than the long form. Indeed, the transporter knockout mice exhibit increased anxiety- and depressive-like behaviors. In the converse experiment, transgenic mice were made that produce more serotonin transporter than normal mice. This resulted in animals that exhibit *reduced* anxiety-like behaviors. These effects of genetic manipulation of transporter levels up and down are very likely due to alterations of brain *development* rather than simply to changes in transporter function in the adult. We know this from experiments involving treatment of normal mice with an SSRI during early development, which yields adult mice with *elevated* anxiety- and depressive-like behaviors. That is, the SSRI has opposite effects on very young mice compared to its effect on adult mice. Recall that administration of SSRIs to adult mice *diminishes* anxiety- and depressive-like behaviors, as it does in human patients.

Unlike the serotonin transporter, serotonin *receptors* do not remove serotonin from the synapse; they are activated by serotonin, and so they mediate the action of this neurotransmitter. The situation is not simple, however, as there are at least 14 different types of serotonin receptors. One of the first to be genetically manipulated was the type 1B receptor, which is involved in the regulation of mood. For instance, a set of molecules that artificially *activate* this receptor are termed *serenics* because they have anti-aggressive, calming effects in both humans and mice. Based on this information, it was predicted that knocking out this receptor in mice should have the opposite effect from the serenics. Indeed, the type-1B knockout mice are hyperaggressive, attacking intruders much more viciously than do normal mice. Interestingly, these knockout mice also display more immobility in the forced swim test, a depressive-like behavior.

Another interesting subtype is serotonin receptor 7. Considerable evidence implicates this receptor in the three linked phenomena of circadian rhythm, sleep, and mood. In assays of depressive-like behavior, knockout mice lacking receptor 7 display reduced immobility time. The same effect is seen using administration of drugs that block receptor 7. Interestingly, SSRI treatment may reduce the level of receptor 7 in the brain. Moreover, combining SSRI treatment with a drug that blocks receptor 7 has a synergistic effect. That is, if low doses of both drugs, which have no effect on behavior at those doses, are combined, a behavioral effect is observed. In the depression model of chronic unpredictable mild stress, the level of serotonin receptor 7 is increased, and this change is inhibited by treatment with the SSRI fluoxetine (Prozac). There are also disturbances in sleep patterns in the receptor 7 knockout mice. These patterns are similar to those observed when SSRIs are administered, and are opposite of the patterns seen in depressed patients. That is, SSRIs in the knockout mice lead to sleep patterns that would be expected for patients who are effectively treated by medication. Collectively, these findings highlight the serotonin type 7 receptor as playing an important role in major depressive disorder. It is also interesting that several antipsychotic medications that are effective in treating schizophrenia bind to the type 7 receptor.

Genetic Mouse Models of Features of Schizophrenia or Autism

As mentioned in the previous chapter, mutations in a number of genes have been identified as candidates for increasing the risk of schizophrenia. However, mutations in most of these candidate genes confer very small effects on the risk for schizophrenia. The gene called *disrupted in schizophrenia 1* (*DISC1*) is an exception to this generalization. The exceedingly rare families in which this gene is disabled display a very high frequency of inherited psychiatric illness. Mutations in DISC1 do not just cause schizophrenia, however; they also cause major depressive disorder and bipolar disorder in different family members. There is also some evidence from other genetic studies implicating DISC1 in autism. Nonetheless, the dominant effects of its mutations in causing mental illness make DISC1 an attractive gene to manipulate in mouse models. One can also imagine future gene therapy experiments in humans, aiming to replace the mutant DISC1 gene with the normal gene.

Some of the transgenic and mutant mouse models that have been made thus far involve inducing the expression of a mutant form of the human DISC1, or blocking the expression of the normal mouse DISC1 gene, or mutating the mouse DISC1 gene. Blocking DISC1 expression in the fetal brain reveals that this gene is critically important for the migration of immature neurons to their appropriate location during embryonic development. This finding supports the premise that mental illness has its origin in the fetus. Introducing mutations into different parts of the DISC1 gene results in mice with either schizophrenia-like or depression-like behavioral abnormalities. Consistent with these results, antipsychotic medications that are effective in schizophrenia attenuate the former symptoms, while antidepressant medications attenuate the latter symptoms in these two different mouse models. These results are consistent with the finding in the families with the DISC1 mutation, where it can lead to schizophrenia, major depressive disorder, or bipolar disorder. These experiments also demonstrate that medications that work in humans can have similar effects on analogous behaviors in mice, supporting the idea that new medications for these conditions can effectively be developed in mice for eventual testing in humans.

It is also relevant that the DISC1 protein was found to interact with the protein GSK3b. This protein is a known target of the medication lithium chloride, which is commonly used to treat bipolar and major depressive disorders. It is clear from just this one example that much can be learned from modeling mutations of psychiatric diseases in mice.

In the case of autism, there are many genes and mouse models to consider. One interesting example is the family of *neuroligins*, which are proteins that are important for the development of synapses. Several mutations in the genes for neuroligin-3 and -4 are found in individuals with ASD. Although only a tiny number of cases with these mutations have been found thus far, they support the hypothesis that dysfunction of synapses is a critical part of the development of autism. That hypothesis is not too much of a stretch, of course, since synapses are the primary method of communication in the brain, and disruption of their functions should lead to all sorts of disorders. In the case of neuroligin 4 mutations associated with ASD, the gene is disabled. Thus, to make a mouse model of this condition, the neuroligin 4 gene was genetically disabled. The neuroligin 4 knockout mice were indeed found to display two of the core features of autism: deficits in reciprocal social interaction and in communication. The latter function was inferred from tests of the USVs of pups separated from their mothers. On the other hand, these knockout mice do not display other features of autism, such as repetitive behavior, anxiety, seizures, or deficits in prepulse inhibition or learning. The lack of these abnormalities, however, is consistent with the results of testing the patients with neuroligin 4 mutations. Recall that these patients were characterized as having ASD and not classical autism. Therefore, it appears that the knockout mice display features of ASD that are consistent with some of the expectations from the human neuroligin 4 mutations.

Modeling Environmental Risk Factors for Schizophrenia and Autism in Rodents

Although it is often stated that no causes of schizophrenia or autism have been identified, a number of environmental factors have repeatedly been shown to have a significant impact on the risk for these disorders. For schizophrenia, these include being born in the winter or spring months, being born and raised in an urban environment, or being born to a mother who experienced severe stress during pregnancy. There are other risk factors as well, but the ones cited here are also consistent with the maternal infection risk factor that was described in the previous chapter. That is, infections are more likely in the fall and winter and in urban environments. Moreover, as described below, stress during pregnancy can evoke some of the same cytokines that are induced during the response to infection. Given the strength of evidence connecting maternal infection with schizophrenia, many investigators are studying this risk factor in mouse and rat models. The goals are to determine if schizophrenia-like neuropathology and behaviors can be found in the offspring of infected mothers, and if so, what molecular mechanisms are responsible for those effects? How does maternal infection alter fetal brain development? Can potential therapeutic interventions be tested? In addition, is it possible to use mice to study how maternal infection interacts with genetic variants that increase susceptibility to schizophrenia?

Several methods are used for studying maternal infection in rodents. The most direct approach (though not necessarily the easiest) is to give a pregnant mouse a flu infection by applying influenza virus to the nasal passages. The mouse displays sickness behavior for several days: she has a ruffled, unkempt fur coat and sits in a corner of the cage with a humped back, moving little. After she recovers, she gives birth and raises her pups. Hossein Fatemi at the University of Minnesota studies these offspring, as does our own laboratory, as young pups, as adolescents, and in maturity as adults.

Our group and that of Ina Weiner at Tel Aviv University in Israel developed a second approach to study the maternal infection risk factor; that method involves injecting a pregnant mouse or rat with a molecule that the immune system recognizes as a virus. This is a synthetic RNA polymer called poly(I:C). The maternal immune system is "fooled" into responding as if there is a viral infection, despite the fact that there is no pathogen present. We refer to this model as *maternal immune activation* (MIA). A third approach is to inject the mother with a different molecule, lipopolysaccharide (LPS), which is a component of bacterial cell walls. This fools the immune system into responding as if there is a bacterial infection. Because the molecular pathways in immune cells that are stimulated by viruses and bacteria have considerable overlap, the results of flu infection and injection of poly(I:C) or LPS are rather similar. Some of these experiments use mice and others use rats; each species has advantages for research. Mice can be manipulated genetically with relative ease, whereas rats are preferred for electrophysiology studies because their larger brains make for easier placement of microelectrodes. The findings of MIA studies are strengthened by the fact that very similar results are obtained with mice and with rats. The offspring of infected or poly(I:C)-treated mothers display neuropathology that is characteristic of schizophrenia and also neuropathology that is characteristic of autism. For instance, the enlarged ventricles characteristic of schizophrenia are present in MIA offspring, and in our laboratory, Limin Shi found that the deficit in Purkinje cells of the cerebellum that is characteristic of autism is also present in these offspring. The group of Urs Meyer and Joram Feldon at the Swiss Federal Institute of Technology in Zurich also found a deficit in brain sections stained to detect the protein parvalbumin. The parvalbumin deficit is prominent in schizophrenia but has also been described in a mouse model of the autism candidate gene *neuroligin 3*. It is not surprising that hallmarks of each disorder are found in the same offspring, given that maternal infection is a risk factor for both disorders, as we saw in chapter 5.

In terms of behavior, our group showed that maternal infection and MIA offspring display reluctance to enter the center of an open field (figure 6.3), which is taken to be a sign of enhanced anxiety under mildly stressful conditions. These offspring also exhibit deficits in prepulse inhibition. Natalia Malkova and I also find that male pups from immune-activated mothers display a lower rate of USVs compared to pups born to saline-injected mothers. In addition, analysis of song structure reveals differences in the repertoire of calls emitted by the pups from MIA versus control mothers. Moreover, as adults, the males from poly(I:C)-injected mothers show significantly fewer USVs in response to a female mouse stimulus. These males also display a deficit in the social interaction test in which they are given a choice between interacting with another mouse and spending time in an empty chamber or a chamber with a novel object rather than a novel mouse. In sum, these results suggest that maternal immune activation yields males with poor social and communicative behavior, which are cardinal symptoms of autism. A predominance of

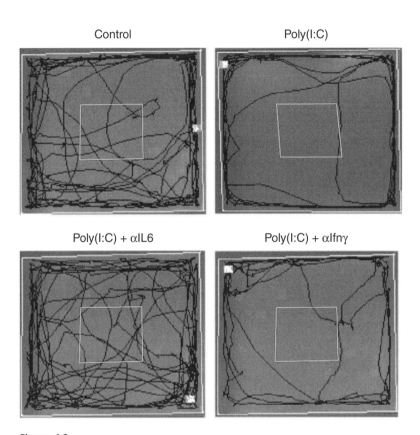

Figure 6.3
Open-field behavior of the adult offspring of poly(I:C)- or saline-treated (control) mothers is illustrated by the lines tracing the movements of individual mice during a 5-minute period. The poly(I:C) offspring are clearly reluctant to enter the center of the field, suggesting enhanced anxiety. In contrast, the offspring of mothers treated with both poly(I:C) and an antibody against the cytokine IL-6 (αIL6) behave like control offspring, showing that the antibody blocks the effects of maternal immune activation. As a control for the general effects of injecting an antibody, an antibody against another cytokine, interferon gamma (Ifnγ), was injected along with poly(I:C), and no effect on the behavior of the offspring is observed. (From Smith et al., 2007)

symptoms in male rather than female mice is also consistent with autism, which occurs much more frequently in males.

As mentioned above, the MIA offspring have other features that are more characteristic of schizophrenia. For instance, several of the behavioral abnormalities manifest only at maturity; adult onset is characteristic of schizophrenia and not autism. In addition, several of the behavioral deficits can be attenuated by treatment with the antipsychotic medications that are used to treat schizophrenia. As mentioned in the previous chapter, the difference in disease outcome from human maternal infection (schizophrenia versus autism) could be due to the timing of the infection or to the genetic background of the mother or the fetus. In the animal studies, there is evidence that both of these factors can influence the outcome of maternal immune activation. As was also mentioned in the previous chapter, mutations in the tuberous sclerosis gene that are linked to autism can influence the outcome of MIA in the mouse. Regarding the timing of infection, Meyer and colleagues showed that the types of behavioral abnormalities displayed by the offspring of MIA mothers are dependent on the stage of gestation in which the immune activator poly(I:C) is administered.

How does maternal infection alter fetal brain development? The poly(I:C) mouse model is well suited to investigate the molecular and cellular pathways that mediate the effects of MIA on the fetus. Since cytokines are induced following maternal infections, and these proteins are known to have the ability to influence fetal brain development, our laboratory group undertook to study their role in MIA. In the first experiment, Stephen Smith injected a variety of cytokines into pregnant mice. Just one of these, IL-6, is able to induce changes in the fetal brain that cause the adult offspring to display abnormal behaviors like those seen in the offspring of mothers given an influenza infection. That is, a single injection of this proinflammatory protein has a permanent effect on the brains of the offspring. In the converse experiment, the effects of IL-6 induced in the mother by poly(I:C) were blocked by simultaneous injection of an antibody against IL-6. This inhibition of IL-6 function results in a complete blockade of the behavioral effects of poly(I:C)-induced MIA on the offspring (figure 6.3). Thus, the inflammatory effects of IL-6 are necessary for MIA to alter fetal brain development. It is worth noting that several very diverse environmental risk factors for schizophrenia, including maternal stress, fetal hypoxia, and maternal malnutrition, as well as maternal infection, are known to induce IL-6. This suggests the possibility that these disparate risk factors could ultimately work through a common pathway that involves inflammation.

Where is IL-6 acting? Also in our group, Elaine Hsiao has identified cells that respond to the IL-6 increases induced by maternal poly(I:C) injection. Responding cells are found in both the fetal brain and the placenta. Thus, IL-6 may have direct effects on neurons in the brain, but also alters the nutritive functions of the placenta. Also important is that the IL-6 induced in the mother by poly(I:C) induces the production of more IL-6 in both the placenta and fetal brain; this increase in local production of IL-6 suggests that a proinflammatory, self-reinforcing, feed-forward cycle may be set up in both tissues by maternal immune activation. Indeed, working with Kim McAllister's group at the University of California at Davis, we find evidence of altered cytokine levels in the blood and brains of fetal, early postnatal, and adult MIA offspring. If this turns out to be relevant for the human situation, it could help explain the state of immune activation seen in the brain and blood of adult patients with schizophrenia and autism that is described in the following chapter.

The key role of inflammation in this paradigm was further demonstrated by Meyer and colleagues, who inhibited inflammation by raising the level of the anti-inflammatory cytokine IL-10 in the poly(I:C) model. This intervention resulted in the blockade of the effects of MIA on the subsequent behavior of the offspring. The successful outcome of blocking inflammation using the anti-inflammatory cytokine IL-10, or an antibody against the pro-inflammatory cytokine IL-6, raises the possibility of intervening in human maternal infection. Could injection of IL-10 or the anti–IL-6 antibody be tested in pregnant women who are experiencing a severe infection? Recall, however, from chapter 3 that a balance of inflammatory events is critical for a normal pregnancy outcome. This means that manipulation of the inflammatory balance in humans may be difficult and even dangerous for the fetus. In fact, in the mouse model, raising IL-10 levels during pregnancy in the *absence* of MIA results in negative effects on offspring behavior. This shows that tipping the balance too far toward the anti-inflammatory side may be as dangerous and tipping it toward inflammation.

Another approach to therapeutic intervention was taken by Ina Weiner and colleagues in Tel Aviv. They manipulated the offspring of poly(I:C)-injected mothers during adolescence, before the onset of some of the behavioral abnormalities and before the onset of some key neuropathology. Specifically, they injected adolescent offspring for a brief period with the antipsychotic medication clozapine, which is used to treat schizophrenia, and then assessed those offspring in later adulthood. The findings are striking: the hallmark of schizophrenia neuropathology, enlarged ventricles, does not develop in the offspring. Moreover, this preventative, antipsychotic drug treatment also averts the adult onset of several of the abnormal behaviors that are induced by maternal immune activation. In addition, this experiment has been successful in both mouse and rat MIA models.

These results highlight the controversial issue of whether those adolescents known to be at very high risk for developing schizophrenia should be treated before the onset of psychosis. This group is identified by symptoms such as paranoia, delusions, or social withdrawal, and possibly by having a family member with the disorder. However, only 30% to 50% of these adolescents will go on to develop psychosis, so a large proportion of the at-risk group would unnecessarily be given a drug that could have unintended effects on brain development. The fact that only a fraction of the at-risk group will go on to become psychotic makes testing drugs in this population problematic. Aside from the obvious ethical considerations, the signal-to-noise ratio for even an effective drug would be expected to be small. This may explain some of the negative results that have so far been obtained in clinical trials testing antipsychotic medications for prevention of schizophrenia in the at risk population. What is needed is a more specific biological marker of individuals who will indeed go on to develop the disorder. If such a marker can be developed, the dramatic results of adolescent antipsychotic medication in the rodents may compel further testing of this prevention strategy in humans. It will also be worth testing in a monkey model of maternal infection. Christopher Coe, at the University of Wisconsin, has recently shown that the offspring of influenza-infected pregnant monkeys display some abnormal behaviors; using MRI analysis of their brains, Coe has also found signs of neuropathology. It should be noted, however, that a study involving administration of anti-psychotic medication to healthy monkeys reported a reduction in the size of the brains. An alternative treatment of at-risk human subjects did show promise in a preliminary double-blind trial. Twelve weeks of treatment with an omega-3 polyunsaturated fatty acid supplement reduced the progression to psychosis by 23%, measured 40 weeks later. Given that this supplement is generally regarded as beneficial to health and without side effects, treatment during the at-risk period is well worth following up.

In summary, it is indeed possible to model both environmental and genetic risk factors for schizophrenia and autism in animals. A variety of animals can exhibit features of these disorders; they can serve as models for the study of the mechanism of disease development and even for testing treatments. Moreover, studies using the maternal infection model provide hints that an inflammatory cascade may be set up in the prenatal offspring, which could lead to inflammatory events in the postnatal offspring. In fact, there is considerable evidence that the immune status of individuals with autism or schizophrenia is strikingly and permanently altered. That evidence is discussed in the next chapter.

7 Immune Involvement in Autism, Schizophrenia, and Depression

For the first time, our chemistry is sophisticated enough that we can take control of the machine that has been keeping us alive, the immune system
—Kary Mullis

We learned in chapter 2 that there are relationships between the brain and immune system at a number of levels. The brain can influence immune function, as happens during depression. The immune system can influence behavior, as happens during peripheral infection when we get a cold or the flu. Proteins produced in the brain, such as MHC, complement and cytokines, are also used by the immune system. The question for this chapter is, could the immune system, or the brain's own immune-related proteins, be involved in autism, schizophrenia, and depression?

Immune-Related Abnormalities in Autism

A significant problem for efforts to learn about the neuropathology of autism is the small number of postmortem brains available for investigators to study. For a brain to qualify for study, the medical history of the subject who died must be well documented, the subject must have died of a cause that does not damage significant parts of the brain, and the postmortem interval (the time between death and removal and preservation of the brain) must be as short as possible. These issues, plus the relatively recent realization of the importance of making such brains available to investigators, have severely limited the study of autism neuropathology. Thus, it was not until 2005 that Carlos Pardo (see box 7.1) and colleagues at Johns Hopkins University Medical School published their groundbreaking paper. This study of nine brains from patients with autism used several

Box 7.1
Carlos Pardo-Villamizar

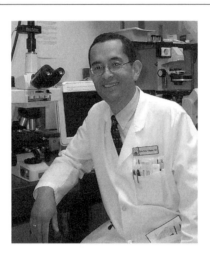

Carlos Pardo-Villamizar's work has focused on neuroimmunological and infectious disorders of the nervous system, including multiple sclerosis, HIV infection, and neurological complications of autoimmune disorders. He also has a strong interest in autism. In fact, his 2005 paper revealed for the first time the strong signs of an inflammatory state in the autistic brain. A surprising and important feature of these data was the striking elevation of cytokines in the cerebral spinal fluid of autistic subjects. Such samples are exceedingly rare in this clinical literature, and were collected by his colleague Andrew Zimmerman. Pardo believes that the genetic and environmental disruption of neuronal connections that lead to autism are magnified by the altered immune status in this disorder.

Pardo's paper brought an immediate and unwanted response: a wave of e-mails regarding the use of autoimmune treatments for autism. In fact, his paper did not present evidence of an autoimmune reaction in the brain. Although his work has opened up a new field of autism research, Pardo is concerned about the misuse of his findings.

We consider premature the use of any immunomodulatory interventions to modify the neuroglial activation and neuroinflammation observed in ASD. Further studies are needed to clarify with better detail the components of the systemic immune and neuroimmune responses. Furthermore, because current treatment approaches to modify neuroimmune responses are nonspecific and may induce more unwanted side effects than benefits, we strongly recommend against the use of any immunotherapy in patients with ASDs until better knowledge of the pathogenic processes is achieved. Current immunomodulatory medications act mostly on adaptive immune system pathways and do not have reliable effects on neuroglial activation or innate immune responses.

Box 7.1
(continued)

Although there are no cures for autism at present, most physicians recommend intensive behavioral therapy and, if asked, warn parents away from experimental treatments. Nonetheless, studies have found that up to three-quarters of families with children who have autism try at least some alternative therapies.

Pardo received his medical degree from Universidad Industrial de Santander in Bucaramanga, Colombia. He obtained training in clinical neurology at the Instituto Neurológico de Colombia in Bogotá. He went on to complete a fellowship in clinical and experimental neuropathology at the Johns Hopkins University School of Medicine. Now an associate professor of neurology and pathology at Johns Hopkins, Pardo is continuing his work on neuroimmunology and sees patients at the Johns Hopkins Outpatient Center. (Photo courtesy of C. Pardo)

methods to uncover striking evidence of an inflammatory-like condition. Staining of brain sections showed that the microglia, the brain's own cells with immune-like functions, are activated in many autism cases. In comparison to a neurologically typical (or neurotypical) brain, the study also found an increased level of an MHC protein associated with inflammation. The prominent microglial activation raises the possibility of monitoring immune status in the brain by imaging subjects using positron emission tomography (PET) methods. There is a new chemical that binds to activated microglia that can be injected into the circulation and enter the brain, where it is visualized by PET imaging. This is also a promising approach for analyzing inflammation in people in whom other disorders involving brain inflammation, such as Alzheimer's and Parkinson's diseases, are suspected.

A particularly striking finding in the Pardo study was that these various markers of immune activation are present in the youngest of the brains studied (5 years old) as well as in the oldest studied (44 years old). This age range implies that immune activation in autistic brains can begin early in life and that it either persists or oscillates throughout life. Pardo went on to test for cytokines in extracts of the brains and found that a number of them, particularly IL-6, were strikingly elevated in autism. Finally, the same paper included a rare analysis of cytokines in the cerebral

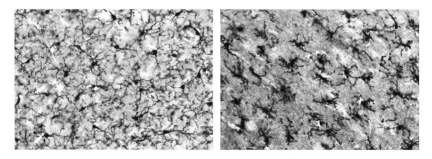

Figure 7.1
Pictures are shown of postmortem brain sections taken from a 15-year-old control (left) and a 14-year-old autistic subject (right). Both sections were stained to visualize microglia, the cells that carry out immune-like functions in the brain. The stained cells in this autism sample display the thick stubby processes that are typical of strongly activated microglia. Other autistic brains in this study show varying degrees of activated microglial cell morphology. Both pictures are of the same magnification. (From Nicole Tetreault)

spinal fluid (CSF) of living autism subjects. High levels of cytokines were observed there also. Recent work by several other groups has confirmed the immune-activated status in many autism cases (figure 7.1) and in a number of brain areas.

Although there is strong evidence of immune activation in the brain in many cases of autism, the condition of these brains does not necessarily imply the presence of an acute inflammatory event. Rather, it appears to represent an ongoing, subclinical condition that may not have been described before, and therefore the evidence merits further study. There are also indications that the degree of immune activation varies widely among the brains tested, which is consistent with the wide range of symptoms seen in autism spectrum disorders (ASD). On the other hand, it could be that immune activation oscillates up and down in the autistic brain, depending, for instance, on life events. This would mean that when a person dies, the brain might be in an activated immune state or a relatively quiescent state.

The fact that the levels of several cytokines such as IL-6 are, on average, strongly increased in autism brain extracts, and that cytokines are also elevated in the CSF of living autism subjects, raises the question of whether these proteins could be actively influencing behavior in a continuous manner. We learned in chapter 2 that the cytokine increases induced by peripheral infection in the body alter behavior by their direct and indirect actions on the brain. This is consistent with animal experiments showing that cytokine injections into the circulation can drastically alter behavior. Moreover, the clinical trials of cytokine injection for cancer treatment revealed that some cytokines cause severe depression in many patients, and even occasionally psychosis. These experiments involve injection into the circulation, and it would be expected that elevated cytokines within the brain itself and in the CSF in autism would have more dramatic effects than those in the peripheral circulation.

The fact that cytokines are elevated in the CSF raises the possibility of using their presence in the fluid as a measure to monitor the immune status of the brain in autistic children. Although invasive, making a spinal tap is a relatively safe procedure to obtain CSF, and it provides information that is much closer to the brain than a blood sample. It has been difficult, however, to establish a proper comparison of the cytokine levels in the CSF of children with autism versus controls—that is, typically developing children of the same age—because research purposes alone do not justify making spinal taps on healthy children. The speculation that cytokines in the brain and CSF in autism have an ongoing influence on behavior is consistent with a small but intriguing study led by Andrew Zimmerman and colleagues at the Kennedy Krieger Institute and Johns Hopkins Medical School. They asked, in autistic children, what are the behavioral effects of being sick with a cold or the flu? In this case, parents filled out a questionnaire that graded a variety of autistic behavioral characteristics. They did this for their children during sickness (objectively measured by fever), and following the end of the fever. The general finding was that autistic behaviors such as irritability, inappropriate speech, and repetitive movements, *decrease* during sickness, but they return after the sickness episode is over. The improvement did not correlate with the degree of lethargy, so the investigators concluded that the results represent a genuine improvement in autistic symptoms.

Among the several possible interpretations of these results, one is that the actual rise in brain temperature during fever alters the electrical firing of certain neuronal circuits, which resulted in normalized behavior. This is not a far-fetched idea; the activity of neuronal circuits is known to be influenced by temperature. Another possible interpretation is that the increase in cytokines elicited by the infection alters the already abnormal balance of cytokines in the autistic brain, tipping it back toward the normal condition. That is, perhaps the cytokine balance is tipped one way in autism, but the set of cytokines induced by sickness happens to tilt the balance the other way. This could result in a transient normalization of behavior. Since the autistic brain exists in an immune-activated state, and getting a cold activates the immune system, the interaction between the two states is predicted to be complex. Investigation using animal models should shed light on this interaction. Regardless of the explanation, this phenomenon deserves further study. Some parents actually report taking their autistic child out to crowded malls in hopes that he will catch a cold, so that they can interact more normally with him for a few days before he recovers.

Another type of investigation lends independent support to the findings of immune activation in autism. The state of activation of nearly all the genes in the brain can be monitored by assaying the level of their corresponding RNAs. Recall that the more RNA made from a gene, the more of its protein product there will be to carry out the functions of the gene. Karoly Mirnics (Vanderbilt University, Nashville) and Antonio Persico (Campus Bio-Medico, Rome) and colleagues did this type of analysis with a set of postmortem autism brain extracts, and compared the data to a set of brain extracts from age-matched controls. They found that, in contrast to those in the neurotypical controls, many immune-related genes were in an activated state in the autism brains. Moreover, these activated genes are known to be associated with the recovery phase of autoimmune brain disorders. Could this permanent state of immune activation represent a response to an early autoimmune attack on the brain?

The latter notion is consistent with results from several laboratories that report the presence in the blood of autistic subjects of antibodies that bind to proteins found in the brain. This suggests the presence of an anti-brain, autoimmune ("anti-self") condition, which could reflect a previous exposure to an antigen, possibly as a result of an injury or other brain insult such as an infection. As discussed in chapter 2, such an immune reaction could be due to molecular mimicry, in which the immune system detects a foreign protein and makes antibodies against it that happen to cross-react with a similar protein in its own brain. It should be emphasized that such antibodies can also be found in blood from control subjects and from patients with various other diseases. However, it has been reported that the amount of such antibodies is higher in some autistic subjects than in control subjects. Normally, such proteins are thought not to be able to enter the brain itself. Can these antibodies actually cross the cellular barrier that separates the blood and the brain and enter the brain? If they do, what effects might they have in the brain?

Because anti-brain antibodies have also been observed in the serum of mothers of autistic children more often than in sera from mothers of typically developing children, David Amaral and colleagues at the University of California at Davis are investigating this phenomenon in a nonhuman primate model. They are asking whether autoimmune antibodies in the circulation of mothers could affect the development of the monkey fetuses. In this experiment, antibodies are purified from the blood of mothers who have had autistic children, as well as from the blood of mothers who have had typically developing children. These different sets of antibodies are then injected into the circulation of pregnant monkeys, and the behavior of the subsequent offspring is assessed for the possible presence of autism-like symptoms. Preliminary results show that some of the offspring of monkeys receiving autism-related antibodies display highly repetitive, stereotyped behaviors. These behaviors are not seen in the offspring of monkeys receiving antibodies from women with typical children. This result suggests that there might be an autoimmune reaction in the mother that affects fetal brain development. It is known that maternal antibodies cross the placenta (which is important for the establishment of initial infant immunity). In fact, there is evidence that the injected antibodies can actually bind to cells in the fetal brain.

A possibly related situation has been found in the autoimmune disease *systemic lupus erythematosus* (SLE, often called lupus). In addition to a wide variety of peripheral symptoms, many SLE patients exhibit cognitive impairment, which is often manifested as a memory deficit. The autoimmunity in SLE is mediated by antibodies, a subset of which bind to receptor proteins on neurons in the brain. Betty Diamond and colleagues at the Columbia Medical Center in New York showed that such antibodies taken from the serum of SLE patients, or from an extract of postmortem SLE brain, can, when injected into mice, kill neurons and cause memory impairment. In order for these effects to occur in adult mice, however, the blood-brain barrier, which normally keeps proteins out of the brain, must be transiently opened. This can be done by injection of lipopolysaccharide, a mixture of bacterial cell wall components that can induce an inflammatory reaction in mice. In an alternative mouse model, the same type of auto-antibodies were evoked in pregnant mice. The offspring of such mice display brain neuropathology as well as striking deficits in learning and memory. These results are consistent with findings that children born to mothers with SLE show a high incidence of learning disorders, while those born to fathers with SLE do not. These human and animal studies suggest that maternal antibodies can be a cause of neuropathology and cognitive impairment.

Auto-antibodies are also thought to be responsible for the childhood disorder *Sydenham's chorea* (previously known as Saint Vitus' dance). The motor symptoms of this disorder—uncontrolled movements in all limbs and facial muscles—as well as psychiatric symptoms such as obsessive-compulsive disorder (OCD), follow some months after a childhood streptococcus infection, as in strep throat or scarlet fever. Antibodies that bind to neurons in the brain are found in this disorder, and these antibodies also bind the strep bacteria, an example of molecular mimicry. The neurons that the antibodies recognize are in the *basal ganglia*, an area of the brain known to control movement. A related syndrome, *PANDAS* (pediatric autoimmune neuropsychiatric disorders associated with streptococcal infections), can follow a strep infection also, but the symptoms (no chorea, but OCD and/or tics as in Tourette's syndrome) appear much sooner after the infection. While the diagnosis of PANDAS as a separate syndrome is controversial, it is interesting that Mady Hornig and Ian Lipkin at Columbia University have used autoimmune-susceptible mice to show that immunization with strep induces antibodies found in the blood and brain that bind to both the bacteria and to neurons. These mice display some repetitive behavioral features reminiscent of OCD.

With regard to autism, additional evidence for an autoimmune connection comes from epidemiologic studies. Although the results are not always consistent across studies, the largest studies have found that children with ASD are more likely than controls to have a family member with an autoimmune disease or allergy. This association appears to be strongest when such a disorder is found in the mother. That is, if a woman has a history of asthma or allergy, or an autoimmune disease such as rheumatoid arthritis or celiac disease, it approximately doubles the likelihood that her child will have autism or ASD. There are several reasons why results can differ among such epidemiologic studies: some cohorts include just autism subjects, while others may include ASD and/or Asperger subjects (a high-functioning ASD group). In addition, the presentation of autism is strikingly heterogeneous, including variable and possibly confounding symptoms such as gastrointestinal (GI) disorders, sleep disorders, epilepsy, mental retardation, and even self-injurious behaviors.

Consistent with an altered autoimmune status are findings from studies of variants of MHC genes in autism families. A great many variants of these genes are found in human populations, and certain variants are more frequent in autistic children as well as mothers of autistic children. One of the variants linked to autism is frequently associated with autoimmune disorders such as rheumatoid arthritis. It is possible that this MHC variant predisposes the bearer to unusual immune reactivity to environmental toxicants or microbes.

In keeping with the epidemiology, there is a general consensus among investigators that abnormalities in the peripheral immune system are present in autism, although there is little agreement on the details. A large, recent study by Paul Ashwood and Judy Van de Water at the University of California at Davis concluded that a number of cytokines are elevated in young ASD children. It also appears that immune cells in the blood of some ASD subjects display a stronger cytokine response to immune stimulation than do cells from control subjects. This is of interest because such hypersensitivity could help explain the initiation and perpetuation of autoimmune responses in some ASD subjects. Another study reported that this hypersensitivity is most prominent in ASD patients who have associated GI symptoms. Of course, the latter result raises the issue of whether the abnormal immune system causes problems for the gut, or if the gut inflammation stimulates the immune system. The same issues apply to the immune activation observed in the brain. Since the brain's own immune-like cells, the microglia, were originally derived from the peripheral immune system, is the latter system ultimately responsible for the brain immune activation? Conversely, could the initial immune activation arise in the brain and then be communicated to the periphery via the neural pathways discussed in chapter 2? Yet another possibility is that the peripheral immune, GI, and brain immune related abnormalities are all driven in parallel by a common stimulus.

For instance, Pat Levitt, now at the Keck School of Medicine at the University of Southern California, found that the presence of a common variant of the gene MET increases the risk for ASD. Levitt also found that the MET protein is reduced in autism brain samples. The key point for the present discussion is that the MET gene is known to play a role in neuronal development and in the GI tract, and is also important in immune system function! Similarly, using the maternal infection mouse model, our group (experiments led by Elaine Hsiao) and that of Sarkis Mazmanian at Caltech showed that, following maternal immune activation in mice, the adult offspring display abnormalities not only in brain development but in the GI system as well. In addition, lymphocytes from the blood of the adult offspring from immune-activated mothers display striking increases in IL-6 secretion when immune-stimulated. The increases are stronger than those seen in lymphocytes taken from control offspring. This hypersensitivity is reminiscent of findings in immune cells from autistic subjects. Thus, a single gene variant (of MET) or a single environmental insult (maternal infection) can have permanent effects on all three systems—brain, GI, and immune.

Hygiene Hypothesis

There has been a dramatic increase in the incidence of allergies, asthma, and autoimmune disease in the past 50 years, and the change has occurred primarily in wealthy, industrialized nations. One hypothesis to explain this discrepancy between developed and third-world countries is that the populations of the wealthy nations have better access to antibiotics and vaccines, and also have improved hygiene and cleanliness inside homes and workplaces. This improved public health very likely *decreases* stimulation of the immune system and reduces the frequency of infections. Of course, exposure to pollutants or pollen, etc., can *stimulate* the immune system and exacerbate allergies. However, it is reasoned that the lack of exposure to pathogens in *infants* restricts the "education" of the developing immune system. Epidemiology studies have shown, for example, that children living on farms, where they presumably get a strong dose of microbes from the soil, animals, and the air, are less likely to get autoimmune diseases than children growing up in cities. We can imagine a housewife being horrified because her urban apartment doesn't smell clean enough, even if it is spotless. Or an urban mom swooping down on her toddler with an antibacterial wipe after each touch on a jungle gym, and not allowing her infant to explore objects with his mouth.

Stronger evidence comes from closely controlled experiments involving mice that are raised in a germ-free environment. These mice turn out to be more susceptible to induced autoimmune diseases that resemble multiple sclerosis. Moreover, the lack of bacteria in the GI tract leads to a strongly increased response to experimentally induced colitis and its associated GI inflammation. Conversely, as shown by Sarkis Mazmanian at Caltech, boosting the level of beneficial bacteria in the mouse gut can help it fend off experimentally introduced colitis and GI inflammation. These bacteria are normally found in the human GI tract, but the levels vary considerably among different people. This is the idea behind the use of "probiotic" bacteria, which are finding their way into various food items in the grocery store, such as certain yogurts.

The bacteria initially present in the human GI tract come from the mother at birth. The fetus itself is sterile, but a normal vaginal birth coats the newborn with microbes from the mother's birth canal. And in fact, it has recently been reported that babies born by Cesarean section are coated with microbes typically found on the skin of adults. These presumably come from the handling the newborns receive after birth. The effects of such abnormal bacterial colonization on both GI and immune status are largely unknown at present, but studies have indeed linked Cesarean births to increased asthma and allergies in those children. This may be another reason to worry about the very high rates of Cesarean section births in the United States.

Another example of the relevance of GI bacteria for maintaining health is a recent report of "fecal transplantation" as a treatment for a very difficult infection by the bacterium *Clostridium difficile*. In a last-ditch effort to recolonize the GI tract of a patient who was dying of this infection, Alexander Khoruts, a gastroenterologist at the University of Minnesota, delivered a small sample of her husband's stool into the colon of the woman. Within a day her diarrhea vanished and the infection disappeared. Lawrence Brandt, Chief of Gastroenterology at Albert Einstein College's Montefiore Medicial Center in New York, says he has done these "human probiotic infusions" on more than 1500 people, to good effect. It is worth noting that there is a report that *Clostridia* species are found more frequently in fecal samples from autistic children than in neurotypical children. More recent evidence indicates that other bacterial species are more prevalent in autism.

It has been speculated that the immune consequences of improved hygiene may also be a factor in the striking increases in the rate of autism diagnosis over the past decade. More specifically, improved hygiene could increase the frequency of autoimmunity in mothers, which could possibly lead to an overreaction against their embryos (discussed in chapter 3). This could involve the induction of antibodies that react with the fetus, including its brain. A different possibility is that the overreactive maternal immune system could lead to a heightened response to maternal infection, itself a risk factor for autism in the offspring.

Immune-Related Abnormalities in Schizophrenia

There are a number of key parallels between the immune-related abnormalities in autism and those in schizophrenia. For example, as in autism, postmortem analysis of the brains of schizophrenia subjects indicates that numerous genes with immune-related functions are activated and producing RNA. The changes in gene expression observed in brains from schizophrenia and autism subjects show a partial, but important overlap in the genes involved in neuroimmune functions. Mirnics and colleagues conclude that "these commonly observed immune changes may represent a long-lasting consequence of a shared, early life immune challenge, perhaps occurring at different developmental stages and thus affecting different brain regions or yielding distinct clinical phenotypes due to different underlying . . . genetic backgrounds." The idea of a common early-life immune challenge is consistent with the maternal immune activation theory discussed in the previous chapter. Mirnics speculates that maternal infection at different stages of gestation or in the presence of different genetic backgrounds could be responsible for the divergent symptoms of autism and schizophrenia.

The activation of immune-related genes in schizophrenia does not signify an acute infection or brain injury (nor does it mean this in autism). In fact, the clinical history of the subjects whose brains were analyzed rules that out. Rather, the suggestion is that there is a subclinical, permanent condition that merits further investigation. And because it is possible and even likely that the adult schizophrenia subjects in this study experienced some negative life events during adulthood that affected their brain chemistry, just the existence of immune activation is not enough to establish its clinical relevance to the disorder; the evidence discussed below is a necessary adjunct. As mentioned in chapter 5, several recent studies that scanned the entire human genome for variants of genes associated with schizophrenia highlighted an area that includes genes coding for the major histocompatibility complex, or MHC. Other genes whose variants are associated with increased risk for schizophrenia include several genes that code for certain cytokines or cytokine receptors.

Another link between immune irregularities and schizophrenia involves autoimmune disease. As is the case for autism, autoimmune disease is associated with schizophrenia. In fact, a very large study of such links in the Danish medical registry, led by William Eaton of the Johns Hopkins Medical School, found that nine different autoimmune conditions are more frequent in schizophrenia subjects than in controls. Moreover, also echoing the connections found with autism, twelve different autoimmune conditions are more frequent in parents of schizophrenia subjects than in parents of controls. In addition, increased levels of self-reactive antibodies have been reported in the blood and CSF of some schizophrenia subjects. Some of these antibodies can bind to tissue sections taken from brain areas implicated in schizophrenia neuropathology. Thus, the possibility of autoimmune damage caused by molecular mimicry has been raised for schizophrenia in the context of maternal infection as well as in the case of postnatal infections by various viruses.

A further link between schizophrenia and immune dysregulation comes from studies of immune cells in the blood. As with autism, there is some inconsistency in the results, but certain generalizations can be made. For example, the levels of a number of cytokines, including IL-6, are elevated in the blood from schizophrenia subjects compared to blood from control subjects. Another feature of immune cells in schizophrenia is that they tend to be hypersensitive to stimulation. This is consistent with the elevated cytokine levels in serum. It is also consistent with some findings in autism, as well as with results from the offspring of immune-activated mouse mothers.

A final point of interest in the context of immune irregularities concerns the molecular mechanism of action of antipsychotic medications. All of the medications in general use that have efficacy in schizophrenia treatment are known to bind to dopamine receptors. Dopamine is therefore a neurotransmitter of great interest in this disorder, and it is known to function in parts of the brain that are affected in schizophrenia. A general finding is that there is too much dopamine function in the schizophrenia brain, and so blocking its receptor lowers the state of activation of cells expressing this receptor. This is the "dopamine theory of schizophrenia." What is less well appreciated, however, is that this dopamine receptor is also found on immune cells in the blood. Moreover, the antipsychotic medications can also bind and alter the function of the immune cells. This has at least two implications. First, it could be that some of the findings of immune abnormalities in schizophrenia are attributable to the use of these medications. That is, the antipsychotic medications may alter the state of the lymphocytes, making them more sensitive to stimulation. Since these medications are widely used in schizophrenia, this possibility is a recurring complication in this research. Many studies control for such effects, however, by also including patients who are either off these medications or have not yet started taking them. A second implication is that some of the antipsychotic effects of the medications could be due to their effects on immune cells, and not just on cells in the brain. For instance, if these drugs affected the balance of cytokines, could this have effects on behavior? It is a question that could be tested in animal studies.

Immune Involvement in Depression

As mentioned in Chapter 2, there are parallels between sickness behavior and some of the symptoms of depression. Both include anorexia, fatigue, sleep disturbances, anhedonia, and depressed mood. Moreover, both major depressive disorder and the effects of peripheral infection on behavior involve bidirectional communication between the brain and the immune system. There are also parallels between stress and depression in terms of their involvement with the HPA axis. There is now little doubt that the immune system and immune-related molecules are an integral part of the story of major depressive disorder.

The immune system is abnormal in otherwise healthy subjects with depression. Patients' blood shows imbalances in the numbers of the various types of immune cells. There are also increased levels of several protein markers of immune activation in the blood. A key finding is that several proinflammatory cytokines, such as IL-6, are elevated in the blood of depressed patients. Moreover, treatment with antidepressant medications can lower IL-6. Cytokine increases are known to activate the HPA axis, and there is a positive feedback loop within that system that can result in further increases in cytokines, both in the brain and in the blood. Normally, the increase in cortisol caused by stimulation of the HPA axis acts to suppress cytokines, but this mechanism appears to be impaired in major depression. Moreover, there are hints that genetic variants in some genes coding for cytokines are associated with responses to antidepressant medications. For instance, one variant in the IL-1β gene is associated with a poor outcome following such treatment. That is, if you carry this variant, your chances of responding well to the medication are less than if you do not have this variant.

Cytokines could also play a role in the diminished size of the hippocampus that is sometimes observed in major depressive disorder. For instance, in studies using adult rodents, proinflammatory cytokines such as IL-6 can inhibit the production of new neurons and can also promote cell death. Moreover, anti-inflammatory medications can block these effects. In animal models of depression, the lower production of new neurons is correlated with some of the depressive-like symptoms (chapter 6).

But are the cytokine increases observed in depression merely a side effect of the stress, smoking, alcohol abuse, lack of exercise, or other environmental and behavioral factors sometimes associated with depression? Or are they part of the causal network that drives depressive behavior, as is the case for sickness behavior? Perhaps the most impressive evidence comes from experiments in which cytokines are injected into human patients for the treatment of cancer or hepatitis. The purpose of this approach is to alter the immune system so as to kill cancer cells or fight infection. In work led by Andrew Miller at the Emory University School of Medicine, the cytokine *interferon-alpha* (IFNα) was injected repeatedly. A side effect of this chronic cytokine treatment is the development of clinically significant depression in 20% to 50% of patients. These are results from double-blind clinical trials, in which neither the patient nor the doctor treating the patient knows whether IFNα or a placebo is being injected. This undesired side effect of the clinical treatment serves as a direct test of the psychiatric effects of cytokine elevation in humans.

In addition, it appears that at least some of the pathways being activated in the brain by IFNα actually overlap with those involved in idiopathic depression—that is, major depression in which the cause is not known (a designation that encompasses most cases). That is, depression results from activation of specific neural pathways, and studies of brain activity using functional MRI show that injection of IFNα activates areas of the brain that are known to be important in major depressive disorder. The evidence that this overlap in pathways is relevant for depression is that the IFNα-induced depressive symptoms respond to conventional antidepression medications such as selective serotonin reuptake inhibitors (SSRIs) like Prozac. In another type of immune activation, vaccination against typhoid also activates the same brain areas that are known to be important in major depressive disorder. In addition, neural activity in the amygdala, a part of the brain that processes emotional and social information, is attenuated following such a vaccination. This could reflect the reorientation toward self-interest and the lack of sociability that is characteristic of sickness and of major depression. In fact, in some healthy people, vaccination against influenza or *Salmonella* can cause depressed mood, lethargy, and mental confusion. Moreover, the severity of those symptoms can be correlated with the levels of cytokines such as IL-6 in the blood.

These results have potential implications for novel treatments of major depressive disorder. For instance, a large, double-blind clinical trial of a blocker of the receptor for the cytokine *tumor necrosis factor-alpha* (TNFα) was run for the treatment of psoriasis, which is an inflammatory disease that may be autoimmune in origin. One surprising result from this trial was that the subjects who happened to have depression as well as psoriasis, and who received the cytokine blocker, showed significant improvement in their depressive symptoms. This effect was independent of any improvement in the psoriasis, so the subjects' mood was not improved just because their inflammatory disease was alleviated. Thus, an unexpected and striking side effect of this anti-cytokine, anti-inflammatory treatment was an improvement in mood.

Improvement in mood was also found when the same TNFα blocker was tested in patients with rheumatoid arthritis. Moreover, a similar type of unexpected side effect was seen in a clinical trial of an anti-inflammatory drug, rofecoxib (Vioxx), in a large number of patients with osteoarthritis. Whereas 15% of the patients were classified as depressed at the outset of the trial, by the end of the trial only 3% were classified as such.

Can suppressing immune status be beneficial for depression under other circumstances? Several double-blind clinical studies of patients with major depressive disorder found that adding an anti-inflammatory drug such as acetylsalicylic acid (aspirin) or celecoxib to the usual SSRI treatment protocol improved outcome for patients who did not respond well to the SSRI alone. This effect of the combination of medications could be due to an anti-inflammatory effect or to the ability of cytokines to alter serotonin uptake, which is what the SSRIs do. In fact, there is evidence that certain cytokines can alter serotonin levels by activating the serotonin transporter. In addition, injections of IFNα alter the levels of serotonin breakdown products found in the cerebral spinal fluid. Thus, manipulation of cytokine levels in depressed patients could alter chemical transmission between neurons as well as treat brain inflammation. Several studies have associated inflammation and elevated cytokines in major depression with increased risk of suicide in those subjects. This suggests that appropriate experimental manipulation of immune status could have an effect on this tragic outcome of major depressive disorder.

Conversely, what about a return to the Wagner-Juaregg experimental approach of *stimulating* immune status? A variety of results from the group of Michal Schwartz at the Weitzmann Institute in Israel suggest that such stimulation can have beneficial effects. For instance, they have recently provided evidence that vaccination of rats can prevent the depression-like state induced by mild chronic stress in these animals. This vaccination protocol involves injecting a peptide (a small part of a protein) that resembles one found in brain myelin, which stimulates an immune response. The researchers are mindful of the potential for causing an auto-immune disease like multiple sclerosis (MS) in this way. Because of the protocol used, however, these animals do not display signs of MS. The rats that undergo chronic mild stress display depressive-like symptoms such as excessive immobility time in the forced swim test and a reduced preference for sucrose in the anhedonia test. The vaccinated animals, however, do not exhibit such strong depressive-like behaviors after exposure to chronic stress. Moreover, the vaccination also prevents the reduction in new neurons in the adult hippocampus that is usually seen following chronic mild stress.

One interpretation of the current state of the art in this field, where apparently contradictory results have been found regarding immune status and depression, is that there is a critical balance that must be maintained in immune status, and that deviating up or down can be harmful. Moreover, restoration of that balance may be achieved by stimulating or inhibiting immune status, depending on the nature of the disorder and the patient. Indeed, as we shall see, there are many different pieces to the immune puzzle, and—to some extent at least—they can be manipulated individually.

In summary, there is plentiful evidence for involvement of immune-related molecules in autism, depression, and schizophrenia. These disorders are often marked by immune-related abnormalities in the brain and in the peripheral immune system. Specific mechanisms for the effects of such abnormalities on behavior include autoimmune antibodies in the adult brain, as well as such antibodies in pregnant women. Those antibodies could be generated by microbial infection. The cytokines arising from infection are also potential culprits, as described for the maternal infection model in the previous chapter. Genetic susceptibility may also interact with these environmental factors. Another environmental factor that has generated great interest in recent years is vaccination, which is the topic of the next chapter.

8 Pre- and Postnatal Vaccination: Risks and Benefits

Is the nation's spiraling rate of autism caused by mercury in vaccines? With over four thousand cases pending, a trillion dollars at stake, and public trust on the line, a firestorm is sweeping from the halls of science to the boardrooms of Big Pharma to the steps of the Capitol.

—Sarah Bridges

The trouble with the world is not that people know too little, it's that they know so many things that just aren't so.

—Mark Twain

We have learned in the preceding chapters that a variety of immune-related abnormalities occur in schizophrenia and autism, including a state of immune activation in the brain, the cerebral spinal fluid, and the peripheral immune system itself. We have also considered the evidence that maternal infection is a prominent risk factor for both disorders, and that the key to that risk factor is likely to be the maternal immune response to infection. That is, immune activation is an important part of the way that maternal infection increases the risk for these disorders. This was shown clearly in the mouse model by the efficacy of substituting direct immune activation of the mother in place of maternal infection (chapter 6). Since immune activation is also a critical feature of vaccination, it is logical to ask whether vaccination could play a causal role in autism or schizophrenia. There are two developmental stages in which vaccination could be important—during pregnancy and in early childhood. The Centers for Disease Control in the United States, as well as similar bodies in other nations, strongly recommends both types of vaccination, and so we shall consider each in turn.

Maternal Vaccination, Schizophrenia, and Autism

A major worry that women often voice is, "Should I get vaccinated while pregnant?" The biggest issue is with flu vaccination, because the influenza virus mutates and comes back each year as a slightly modified version that may not be neutralized by the previous year's vaccine. Thus, if a woman becomes pregnant just before the new vaccine is ready, she must decide whether to get vaccinated with the new vaccine while pregnant. For the Centers for Disease Control in the United States, there is no doubt: all pregnant women should be vaccinated during the flu season. On the one hand, this recommendation is somewhat surprising, because regulatory agencies consider pregnant women and their fetuses as particularly worthy of special caution, especially during early pregnancy. On the other hand, as discussed in chapter 3, pregnancy involves changes in the mother's immune system such that she is in a "controlled inflammatory state" that can lead, for example, to an exacerbated response to pneumonia. She also has reduced lung capacity and increased cardiac output, particularly late in pregnancy. Thus, a serious respiratory infection, particularly during this later period, could make the mother vulnerable to pneumonia that could threaten the fetus or even the life of the mother.

Prior to 1995, because no increased risk of serious outcome for pregnant women, compared to other healthy women, had been found for seasonal flu infection, the U.S. Advisory Committee on Immunization Practices had not recommended universal immunization of pregnant women. In 1995 the committee altered its policy and recommended immunization during pregnancy, except for the first trimester. In 2004, however, the policy was expanded to recommend immunization at any stage of pregnancy. In Canada, the National Advisory Committee on Immunization also changed its policy in 2004, and recommended vaccination in the third trimester. In 2007, the recommendation was expanded to include universal vaccination of healthy women at any stage of pregnancy. These changes in policy, however, do not appear to have been prompted by truly compelling new evidence regarding the risks or efficacy of the vaccines.

A recent review of the literature by Danuta Skowronski and Gaston De Serres of the British Columbia Centre for Disease Control concluded that [influenza vaccination] protection against serious outcomes in pregnant women has not yet been shown. Although harm has also not been shown, sample size to date is insufficient to assert [vaccine] safety in first trimester. Benefit-risk analysis suggests that [vaccination] may be warranted at any stage of pregnancy during certain pandemics and annually among women with select comorbidities. . . . Evidence is otherwise insufficient to recommend routine [vaccination] as the standard practice for all healthy women beginning in early pregnancy.

"Comorbidities" refers to conditions that may exacerbate the response to flu infection, such as asthma or other respiratory conditions. The phrase "certain pandemics" refers to those rare seasonal viruses that hit pregnant women particularly hard, such as the Spanish flu of 1918, which was said to result in a loss of pregnancy in 26% of infected women. Similarly, the 2009 pandemic targeted young adults and pregnant women to an unusual extent, probably because of its close immunological relationship to the 1918 virus (as described in chapter 1). Given the current state of our ability to characterize viral strains, it is very difficult to predict which seasonal flu viruses will affect pregnant women severely; thus, there is always uncertainty involved in the recommendations made at the outset of the flu season. It is also worth noting that none of the published epidemiologic studies assessing outcomes of maternal influenza vaccination have specifically addressed the risk of schizophrenia or autism in the offspring. Mouse studies of maternal influenza infection provide another piece of the puzzle that is relevant to the issue of safety. Recall from chapter 6 that this infection during mid-gestation, which is equivalent to the first trimester of human brain development, leads to mouse offspring exhibiting abnormal behaviors consistent with those seen in autism and schizophrenia, as well as neuropathologic hallmarks of both disorders. More important for the present discussion, most of these characteristics can be reproduced by simply stimulating the maternal immune system, in the absence of a pathogen; and vaccination, of course, is a form of immune stimulation. The rodent experiments have not yet involved an actual vaccination, however, so the animal model story is not complete.

Other considerations are the degree of sickness caused by infection, and the response of the mother to vaccination. Our experiments with flu infection in mice indicate that the intensity of the infection (i.e., the amount of virus administered and the level of sickness behavior in the mother) can predict the level of abnormal behavior in the offspring. Similarly, the amount of immune stimulant (poly(I:C); see chapter 6) administered to

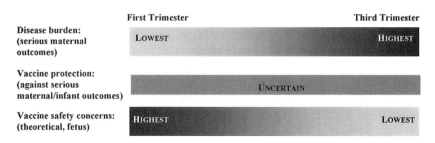

Figure 8.1

For influenza vaccination of pregnant women, there may be gradients during the time of gestation for both infection risk (upper bar) and vaccine safety (lower bar). The most risky stage for infection is likely to be the third trimester, whereas the most risky stage for vaccination is likely to be the first trimester. The timing for optimal vaccine protection is uncertain (middle bar). (From Skowronski and De Serres, 2009)

the mother determines the degree of abnormal behavior in the mouse offspring. This suggests that, all other factors being equal, the severity of infection, and the severity of the maternal reaction to vaccination, will be strong determinants in the outcome for the human fetus as well. Of course, "all other factors" are never equal. Some of the factors likely to play a role include the timing of the infection (see figure 8.1), and the mother's reaction to the vaccine, which will be influenced by the set of genes she carries that regulate her immune responses. If she is prone to respiratory disorders, for instance, her reaction to the vaccine may be more pronounced, just as it would be to the infection itself. The genetic background of the mother, as well as that of the fetus, may also include risk factors for autism or schizophrenia that could influence the outcome. Recall the discussion in chapter 5 about the tuberous sclerosis gene mutations that can cause autism symptoms. In a mouse model of this disorder, activating the immune system of mutant mothers made the symptoms in the offspring more severe than the symptoms in the offspring from an untreated mutant mother, or in the offspring of immune-activated mothers who were not mutant in this gene. Recall also that the *MET* gene, some natural variants of which can increase the risk for autism, plays a role both in fetal brain development and immune system function. Thus, a single gene variant could influence both brain development and the response to infection or vaccination.

The influence of these various factors also helps explain why every woman who experiences an infection during pregnancy does not have a child with autism or schizophrenia. It also seems clear that more research, both in animals and in humans, is needed on both the safety and the efficacy of maternal vaccination.

Early Postnatal Vaccination and Autism

It is probably fair to say that parents are more concerned today about the safety of early childhood vaccinations than ever before. There are many reasons for this. Probably most important is the concurrence in time between a vaccination and the onset of some cases of regressive autism. That is, some parents report that their child was developing normally until a vaccination, after which there was loss of language and social interaction, and the onset of other features of autism. This is the regressive form of autism. Other parents report that the normal linguistic and social development of their child ended following vaccination. A second reason for the increased concern about vaccination is that the connection with autism was elevated to the level of medical discourse by a 1998 publication in the journal *Lancet* by Andrew Wakefield and colleagues, then at Royal Free Hospital in London. They reported on 12 children whose autism symptoms appeared within one month of receiving the MMR (measles, mumps, rubella) vaccine. The authors further claimed to have detected the presence of measles virus in the gastrointestinal (GI) tracts of autistic children but not in children without autism. The autistic children had GI inflammatory symptoms as well. A third and very important factor was that Wakefield's press conference coincident with the publication stimulated the British press to take up this issue in a major way. In the United States too, this story and the stories of vocal and aggrieved parents were widely publicized on television, in the press, and on the Internet. Several famous stars, high-profile politicians, and activists drew further attention to the potential connection between vaccination and autism. Fourth, the number of recommended vaccinations for young children has increased, and the incidence of autism diagnosis has dramatically increased as well. Fifth, there is plenty of precedent for the idea that vaccinations can be dangerous. For instance, a live, attenuated polio vaccine caused paralysis in some recipients, and in the mid-1950s an inactivated polio vaccine caused not only paralysis but some deaths as well. Measles vaccine can cause a bleeding disorder called thrombocytopenia, in about 1 out of every 25,000 vaccinated children. It is estimated that 1 out of 100,000 people who received a swine flu vaccination developed a rare form of paralysis called Guillain-Barré syndrome. A sixth reason for concern is that a preservative in some vaccines, thimerosal, is known to be potentially toxic to the nervous system. Finally, there is widespread suspicion that large pharmaceutical companies will pursue profits over safety. A recent example was Merck's cover-up of the sometimes deadly cardiovascular risks of its blockbuster pain medication Vioxx. Moreover, there has been considerable, well-deserved publicity about medical researchers receiving large fees for speaking on behalf of products of the pharmaceutical industry. Some researchers were even paid large personal fees by companies making the drugs that the same researchers were in charge of testing in clinical studies.

In the face of all of these concerns, is it any wonder that the public is distrustful of exhortations from medical doctors and government agencies that all children should be vaccinated? The most important factor, however, should be the scientific and medical evidence concerning the connection between vaccination and autism. How do the scientific points raised above stand up to close scrutiny?

The Wakefield Paper

The original Wakefield paper has been completely discredited, and there is recent evidence of fraud in the data as well. Ten of the 13 authors subsequently withdrew their names from the publication when they became aware of relevant ethical and scientific issues. The *Lancet* has withdrawn the paper as well. The editor said that if he had known that Wakefield was being paid a large sum of money by a law firm that was preparing to bring suit against the makers of the MMR vaccine, he would not have published the article. In addition, the presence of measles virus in the GI tracts of autistic children was disproved by subsequent and more careful studies. Moreover, because of a number of ethical problems, Wakefield was fired from his position at Royal Free Hospital and subsequently barred from practicing medicine in England. He has also been let go from several subsequent positions in the United States. His explanation for the downturn in his fortunes is that the medical establishment wishes to suppress his findings.

Coincidence in Timing

Regarding the coincidence in timing between MMR vaccination and the onset of autism symptoms or regression, a calculation was done using figures available for England in 1998. Approximately 50,000 children per month received a MMR vaccination between one and two years of age. At the time this calculation was made, the prevalence of autism in England was said to be 1 per 2,000 children. This means that approximately 25 children *per month* would be diagnosed with autism within a month of a MMR vaccination—purely by chance. This extraordinary number means that there will be a great many parents who notice the coincidence in timing between the shot and the symptoms, and some who will be convinced that the connection is causal. Not surprisingly, such parents led the way in the push to have the relationship between vaccination and autism carefully explored by scientific studies.

Epidemiologic Studies

Contrary to some activists' claims, the medical community heard these pleas, took notice of the Wakefield publicity, and conducted a variety of studies to explore the potential connection. As of 2009, 13 epidemiologic studies, generated in a number of different countries, have been published on the subject of autism and vaccination (summarized by Gerber and Offit; see the reading list). Some studies compared the increasing rate of autism diagnosis with the rate of vaccination. Other studies compared the rates of diagnosis of the "new" form of autism proposed by Wakefield—regression with GI symptoms—with the rate of MMR vaccination. Still other studies compared the rates of autism in vaccinated versus unvaccinated children. Another study evaluated the timing of the autism diagnosis in comparison to the MMR vaccination. A different study compared the age at vaccination and the rate of autism. Summarizing these findings, it is fair to say that epidemiologists have been unable to find a connection between MMR vaccination and autism, either the standard type or the proposed "new" type. There is also no effect on the rate of autism and the timing of the vaccination. Moreover, there is no genuine, statistical connection between the timing of the diagnosis and the timing of the vaccination.

    Since there is apparently no connection at the population level, is it possible that there is a subset of autism cases that are driven by vaccination? We know that there is great variability in the range and depth of symptoms in autism. We also know that there is significant variability in the extent of immune activation in samples from autistic brains, cerebral spinal fluid, and blood. These facts are consistent with a hypothesis that there are multiple causes for autism, or that ASD is actually a group of diverse disorders. Epidemiologists argue, however, that since very large sample sizes were evaluated, they have the statistical power to detect small changes—small groups of autistic children whose diagnosis was connected to MMR vaccination. They report no evidence of such subpopulations. Recall that large studies of flu and measles vaccinations could detect adverse effects that occurred in 1 in 25,000 or even 1 in 100,000 cases. Of course, if the subpopulation is extremely tiny, no study could detect it; but then it would not be meaningful in the discussion of potential dangers of vaccination for autism.

Thimerosal

Once such data had emerged, attention turned from the MMR vaccine itself to the potential effects of thimerosal, the antibacterial agent that has been used in some vaccines as a preservative for more than 50 years. Since the MMR and other live virus vaccines did not contain thimerosal, the focus of concern shifted to those vaccines that did. In fact, it made sense to be suspicious of thimerosal because it contains mercury, an agent that is known to be toxic to the nervous system at high doses. The syndrome of mercury poisoning is well known. Although the symptoms of mercury poisoning do not resemble those of autism, the worry is, what effects might mercury have at lower doses? The fact that the U.S. government subsequently banned the use of this preservative added fuel to the fire, raising suspicions that the government had evidence of an autism–thimerosal connection. However, this precautionary move seems to have been long overdue in any case. The removal of thimerosal from vaccines in 1992 in Europe and in 2001 in the United States enabled epidemiologists to compare the rates of autism diagnosis before and after thimerosal removal. The results showed that the rapid rise in autism diagnosis in Europe took place *after* the agent was removed. Another study found that the level of thimerosal exposure (some children received different vaccines with different doses of the agent) did not correlate with the rate of autism. In all, seven major studies of this issue have been published as of 2009. None have found a link between thimerosal exposure and the risk of autism.

Changes in Diagnostic Criteria

A caveat remains, however, that the very large increases in the rates of autism diagnosis may be due to changes in diagnostic criteria or to the drive for social services that impels parents to actively seek an autism diagnosis. Although there are studies indicating that the rise in autism is, in fact, real, what would be the consequences if it were *not* real? If the rise is not due to biological factors, then the thimerosal studies finding no correlation between the rise in autism and the use of the preservative may be invalid. That is, if the rise in diagnosis is due to changes in diagnostic criteria, for instance, then the fact that the rise in diagnosis occurred after thimerosal was taken out of the vaccines is not relevant. Moreover, the expectation that autism diagnosis should drop after thimerosal removal would be invalid as well. On the other hand, if the striking rise in autism diagnosis does not have a biological basis, then the increased number of vaccinations given to children in recent years would be irrelevant as well.

The Number of Vaccinations

What about the increased number of vaccinations now given to individual children? Currently, 14 are given, whereas in 1980 just 7 were given. On the other hand, because of advances in vaccine technology, the number of actual bacterial and viral products (antigens) in today's vaccines total about 200; the total in 1980 was about 13,000. Also relevant is the fact that children are routinely exposed to a truly vast array of antigens during early development, an exposure that is critical for "educating" their immune systems to fight off infections in the future. It is estimated that the average child is infected with 4 to 6 viruses per year (the rate probably depends on the day care center!). Such infections can make the child far sicker than a vaccination. It can be expected, therefore, that vaccinations represent a relatively minor component in the total exposure that the immune system experiences during the first few years of postnatal life.

The GI Connection

Wakefield's 1998 paper presented evidence of an unusual degree of inflammation in intestinal biopsies taken from the autistic children. Unfortunately, this small study suffered from what is known as referral bias. That is, all of these children had been referred to a GI specialist because they had gastrointestinal problems. It was not an actual survey of GI problems in autistic children. Recently, a panel of 28 autism and GI experts was convened to study the issue of GI symptoms in autism. Although they recognized that the available evidence was limited, they concluded that, "the preponderance of data were consistent with the likelihood of a high prevalence of gastrointestinal symptoms and disorders associated with ASD." Thus, such a connection is indeed possible, and merits further study. Moreover, it is logical to expect that the presence of severe GI symptoms would create or exacerbate behavioral problems. The panel of experts also considered the question of diet, and concluded, "Anecdotal reports that restricted diets may ameliorate symptoms in ASD in some children have not been supported or refuted in the scientific literature, but these data do not address the possibility that there exists a subgroup of individuals who may respond to such diets." Here too, more studies are needed.

The issues of diet and GI problems are relevant for the topic of vaccination because all three potentially involve the immune system. Recall from the previous chapter that several researchers have reported increased rates of autoimmune disease and allergies in families with autism. Food allergies can affect GI status, and the incidence of allergies is rising dramatically, at least in developed countries. These observations are also pertinent to the discussion in the previous chapter about the "hygiene hypothesis"—that the increasingly clean environment experienced by children may affect their immune status and susceptibility to allergies. The clean environment may also have an impact on the species composition of the bacteria in the gut. Indeed there have been reports that, compared to samples from typically developing children, the stools of ASD children contain higher levels of potentially toxic bacterial species.

In many cases of schizophrenia, too, there are GI abnormalities. The prevalence of *celiac disease* is higher among schizophrenia patients than in the general population. Celiac disease is an autoimmune disorder that is also linked to autism, depression, and attention deficit hyperactivity disorder. The GI inflammation in celiac disease is the result of an immune reaction to gluten-containing grains, including wheat, rye, and barley, in genetically susceptible individuals. The autoimmune reaction can be detected by tests for certain antibodies, and schizophrenia subjects have 6 to 8 times higher levels of such antibodies than controls. Celiac disease can be distinguished from simple gluten sensitivity by the nature of the pathology. Schizophrenia subjects fall into two groups, those with gluten sensitivity and those with celiac disease; the latter group may be the one that is genetically susceptible. This finding may also be relevant to autism, where gluten sensitivity is commonly reported by parents (although the efficacy of gluten-restricted diets remains to be definitively proven, as noted above).

Benefits of Vaccination

Despite the lack of evidence thus far for a connection between autism and childhood vaccination, history has also shown that vaccinations can be harmful under other circumstances, at least in a very small number of people. Therefore, it is essential to consider what would happen if one or more vaccines where *not* given. That is, what are the benefits of vaccination that need to be balanced against the potential, if unproven in this case, harmful effects? The answer is perhaps less obvious since vaccinations have largely eliminated measles, mumps, and rubella, for instance, as common diseases of childhood in developed nations. Why get vaccinated for diseases that are no longer a threat? Unfortunately, that such viruses can still be a threat is evidenced by the increase in measles seen in populations where not all children are vaccinated. A significant number of unvaccinated children have actually died from measles infections in the United States in recent years, for instance. Congenital rubella infection can cause a series of serious, incurable disorders in the offspring, but this outcome has been virtually eliminated by routine vaccination. An argument used by some parents to justify not vaccinating their children is that the "herd effect" will protect them. That is, when most of the other children are vaccinated, the odds of a measles infection spreading to their own offspring are low. The problem is, of course, that when enough parents make that argument, we no longer have a herd effect. The freedom-of-choice argument is not strong when it comes to public health issues.

This book has dwelled almost exclusively on the dangers of various neuroimmune interactions. It is time, in the next chapter, to discuss some of the experiments and observations that reveal how mental disorders can be prevented and even reversed.

9 Reasons for Optimism

If at first, the idea is not absurd, then there is no hope for it.
—Albert Einstein

Be an optimist, at least until NASA starts moving pairs of animals to the launching pad at Cape Canaveral.
—P. H. Patterson

Preventing or reversing mental disorders—are such notions even plausible? This chapter takes up the challenge of discussing old as well as very recent approaches to these questions.

Disease Prevention

Since genetics make a significant contribution to both schizophrenia and autism, one might guess that the only way to prevent having a child with such a disorder would be to avoid conceiving if there is a person with the disorder in one's family. But, except for rare families and a few very uncommon disorders, these conditions do not display Mendelian inheritance. That is, the chance of having a child with the disorder is very small even if the disorder has appeared in one's family. Moreover, recent genetic studies have presented evidence that some fraction of the incidence of schizophrenia and autism is due to spontaneous mutations— mutations that appeared for the first time in the fetus and are not inherited from the parents. How large this fraction is will be determined by ongoing research.

In chapter 5 we learned that environmental factors in play a significant role in these disorders. For instance, we reviewed the considerable evidence that maternal infection is linked to schizophrenia in the offspring. But just how important is this risk factor? Colds and flu are extremely common, but only about 1% of the population has schizophrenia. Thus, it is obvious that not all children of infected women go on to become schizophrenic. From the various epidemiologic studies cited in chapter 5, it is possible to estimate the frequency of the disorder in the offspring of mothers who experienced such infections during pregnancy. Alan Brown's estimate is that approximately 15% to 20% of the cases of schizophrenia in his cohort of subjects would not have occurred if influenza infection had been completely avoided. This type of calculation is termed "attributable proportion of risk" or "population attributable proportion," and it takes into account the number of people exposed to the risk factor and the likelihood that an individual will get the disorder when exposed to the risk factor. For example, if smoking caused lung cancer in every person who smoked, but only a tiny fraction of the population smoked, the attributable proportion of risk would be small. The same conclusion would hold if the risk to the individual was small but a large fraction of the population smoked. In the case of schizophrenia, the fact that influenza infections are very common raises the attributable proportion of risk. Brown's calculation of 15% to 20%, if accurate, would clearly signify that a sizable proportion of schizophrenia cases are attributable to maternal flu infections.

That is not the whole story, however. The calculation becomes even more impressive when one takes into account all of the other maternal infections that increase risk. Since maternal flu, genital infections (herpes, etc.), and *Toxoplasma gondii* (parasite) infections are all risk factors, and the infections are largely non-overlapping, Brown estimates that if pregnant women could be protected from all these infections, approximately 30% of schizophrenia cases could be prevented. Note that even this estimate does not take into account the contribution of maternal bacterial infections, which also convey risk to the fetus.

Another factor should be considered in the calculations of risk. When it is said that exposure to maternal flu infection increases the risk to the fetus three- to sevenfold, the number does not take into account genetic susceptibility. Since genetics play a significant role in schizophrenia, it is reasonable to assume that some fraction of the populations studied by Brown and other epidemiologists harbor genetic susceptibility for the disorder. Since we cannot presently screen for all of the possibly relevant genes, we also do not know how large that proportion is. Nonetheless, we may assume that a significant fraction of the studied population does not harbor the susceptibility risk genotype, and thus may not become schizophrenic regardless of exposure to relevant environmental factors. The presence of such people would lower the signal-to-noise ratio in the epidemiologic study. Put another way, not being able to subtract out non-susceptible people from the calculations means that, for the subset of people who *do* carry the susceptibility genotype, the risk is probably much higher than three- to sevenfold.

How realistic is it to imagine these infections could be prevented? Does the reality that they are so common mean they are not preventable? In fact, there is nothing mysterious or surprising about the commonsense strategies to avoid such infections. Protection from the parasite *T. gondii*, which is carried to humans by cats or by undercooked meat in the diet, is straightforward: do not handle cat litter or eat raw meat while pregnant. Similarly, the use of barrier protection during sex while pregnant is also straightforward. On the other hand, activation of a latent *T. gondii* infection cannot currently be prevented. Nor is it now possible to prevent activation of latent herpes virus, but the severity of the eruption can be muted by antiviral medications.

The biggest challenge in protecting pregnant women from infection comes from influenza, given its ubiquity during winter months. As discussed in the previous chapter, there are questions regarding the safety and efficacy of vaccination during pregnancy. Certainly, public health agencies strongly recommend such vaccinations, and women who plan on getting pregnant should definitely seek vaccinations. But the advisability of vaccination during the first trimester of pregnancy is still an open issue in the minds of some experts, unless the woman is in a high-risk group for serious complications of infection.

There are a variety of other ways to reduce risk of respiratory infections. Washing one's hands frequently during the day, and using antimicrobial wipes immediately after shopping or putting gas in the car are obvious and easy precautions. In some parts of the world, wearing a mask in crowded public places to avoid spreading or catching an infection is not uncommon. Avoiding airplane trips or wearing a mask during such trips would be sensible for a pregnant woman. A more serious problem is the presence of toddlers at home during pregnancy. Avoiding their frequent infections is not really practical, except by vaccination. Unfortunately, there is no effective vaccination for the common cold at present, although potential vaccines and other medications are under development. Several medications (such as Tamiflu and Relenza) can inhibit the spread of a flu infection within the respiratory system if taken immediately after exposure. These medications are reasonable options; however, we cannot predict their effectiveness against future strains of the virus.

Virtually everyone is aware of these basic precautions, but few people follow them—largely because of a lack of public awareness of the maternal infection risk factor. In fact, when I give lectures on this topic to general audiences, a common response is, "I follow science advances in the newspaper and on TV, but I never heard of this issue before!" In fact, there are striking differences in the coverage of public health issues among countries. When I gave a talk on maternal infection at a scientific meeting in Melbourne, Australia, a few years ago, the local press spread the news and I ended up being interviewed by nine different radio stations and newspapers, including two national newspapers. In contrast, I have never been interviewed for a newspaper article in the United States, despite having given numerous talks at scientific meetings. This might be due in part to the current bias in the United States toward coverage of advances in genetics. ("Genetics envy" is common among researchers in other fields.)

The bottom line is that the risk of many common infections can indeed be significantly reduced—and this extends to the risk for both schizophrenia and autism, as discussed in chapter 5. Another factor in disease prevention is maternal nutrition. Recall from chapter 4 that the risk for several adult-onset diseases is influenced by the health and nutritional status of the pregnant mother. Moreover, malnutrition increases the risk for schizophrenia in the offspring. Specific dietary components may also play a role. Vitamin D, for example, is commonly deficient in women of childbearing age; most of the body's vitamin D comes from exposure to sunlight, which can be limited by a number of environmental and lifestyle factors. John McGrath and his colleagues at the University of Queensland in Australia have provided evidence that vitamin D is important for brain development and that its deficiency may be relevant for schizophrenia.

Consistent with this notion are epidemiologic findings that birth during winter and spring months or in urban areas increases the risk for schizophrenia. Decreased exposure to sunlight could result from either of these environmental factors. There is also an increased risk for schizo-phrenia in the offspring of dark-skinned migrants to countries such as England, where there is relatively little exposure to the sun. In addition, a very recent epidemiologic study in Denmark found that newborns with a low concentration of vitamin D in their blood have an increased risk for schizophrenia as adults. Surprisingly, a high level of vitamin D is also associated with an increased risk. This type of U-shaped risk curve has also been observed in studies of the correlation between vitamin D status and neonatal growth, as well as later cardiovascular disease. These results raise the question of what is the optimal dose for dietary supplements of vitamin D.

Research with an animal model of vitamin D deficiency has provided interesting data. In a rat model of vitamin D deficiency, pregnant animals are fed a diet missing the vitamin, and returned to a normal diet when the pups are born. The adult offspring of such mothers display several behav-ioral abnormalities consistent with those seen in schizophrenia, and they have enlarged ventricles in the brain, a key structural feature of the disor-der. Interestingly, these offspring also display alterations in immune organ morphology and immune cell function. These immune system changes could possibly affect behavior, as discussed in chapter 2. Thus, vitamin D deficiency is another environmental factor that can be manipulated to prevent disruption of brain development, and possibly to lessen the risk of schizophrenia as well. The opportunity to prevent a severely disabling disorder such as schizophrenia with a simple, safe, and inexpensive nutri-tional supplement is a possibility that should be vigorously pursued. There are, of course, many other such dietary factors that influence brain devel-opment, but a connection to schizophrenia or autism has not been firmly established for most of them.

Another common dietary deficiency in pregnancy is choline, an essen-tial nutrient that is used in the biosynthesis of the neurotransmitter acetylcholine and is also an important component of cell membranes. A dietary deficiency in choline can be due to poor nutrition, genetic abnor-malities, or stress (it is directed to the liver for breakdown in the latter condition). The link to the present discussion is due to the work of Robert Freedman and colleagues at the University of Colorado Denver. They have spearheaded studies showing the importance of acetylcholine in schizophrenia. In particular, mutations in one of the receptors for this neurotransmitter are linked to increased risk for schizophrenia. More-over, this receptor is activated by nicotine, and schizophrenia patients are exceptionally heavy smokers. It is thought that such smoking is an uncon-scious attempt at self-medication, as smoking, nicotine, or other drugs that activate this particular acetylcholine receptor do normalize certain symp-toms of schizophrenia, at least temporarily. It is possible that a deficit in dietary choline could lead to lower levels of acetylcholine, which could exacerbate such symptoms. Freedman and colleagues have established a correlation between one symptom, a deficit in what is termed P50 sensory gating, and schizophrenia. Moreover, the acetylcholine receptors linked to schizophrenia are involved in this sensory gating. P50 levels are also cor-related with cognitive function and attention, and deficits in P50 can be ameliorated by drugs that bind and activate this receptor.

Furthermore, this acetylcholine receptor is at its highest levels during fetal brain development. In addition, in animal studies, choline supple-mentation during gestation improves cognition in rats and also improves P50 sensory gating scores in mice that are deficient in this type of acetyl-choline receptor. Because of the possible very early functional role for this receptor, a clinical test was carried out on sleeping infants born to mothers with schizophrenia. P50 gating was measured by electroencephalography (EEG) using wires applied to the skin of the head while the infant is sleep-ing and it was found that the infants in this study displayed, on average, differences in P50 from control infants. Because risk for schizophrenia is higher in families with this disorder, these results suggest that the EEG test may have predictive value for detecting risk for later development of schizophrenia. Given these results, a placebo-controlled clinical trial has begun to test the effect of supplementation of dietary choline in pregnant women and their newborns. Preliminary results indicate that this supple-ment many indeed improve P50 gating in the offspring. Regarding the main topic of this book, it is worth noting that choline supplementation may also suppress inflammation, as activating this acetylcholine receptor clearly has such a function. Choline can activate this receptor either directly, by binding to it, or indirectly, by increasing the level of acetyl-choline. For these reasons, we are currently testing choline supplementa-tion in our mouse model of maternal immune activation to see if this preventive therapeutic approach can reduce schizophrenia-like symptoms in the offspring.

Disease Reversal

Is there any reason to think it might be possible to reverse the symptoms of the disorders we have been discussing—in the young or even adult patient? Once the structure and wiring of brain circuits has been disturbed during early development, is there any hope for intervening later in life? Certainly, the behavioral interventions used currently in autism treatment can be effective, and antipsychotic medications can alleviate some of the symptoms of schizophrenia. Antidepressant medications and psychotherapy are also effective in a subset of severely depressed patients. But just as obvious is the need for more effective treatments. A critical question is, once the symptoms have appeared, is it too late to reverse the neurobiology of these disorders?

There is considerable evidence that brain structure and function is abnormal early on in the course of autism and schizophrenia, and some studies indicate that the same may be true of major depressive disorder. Results from structural MRI studies show that infants who will go on to be diagnosed with autism as toddlers have larger brains than typical infants. This growth then slows below normal levels, so that the size of the brain in autism levels out to approximately normal by adolescence. Neither the cause nor the significance of the early brain overgrowth is understood at this time, but the phenomenon does signal that something is amiss early on. Eric Courchesne and Karen Pierce at the University of California at San Diego have recently found abnormalities in brain function in infants who will go on to be diagnosed with autism. This remarkable study is being done using functional MRI on sleeping infants. That is, they are allowed to fall asleep naturally after being placed in the apparatus. Sounds and voices are played to them, and brain responses are recorded. The key finding is that the autism brain (as later diagnosed) processes this auditory information differently than a neurotypical brain. This is the first objective evidence of altered function at such an early age.

The observation of early differences in brain function is in line with the alterations in behavior that can be detected in children with autism as early as one and a half years of age. It is also consistent with findings from studies of environmental risk factors, such as maternal infection, thalidomide, and valproic acid (discussed below), which indicate that the first trimester of gestation is a key window of vulnerability (see also chapters 5 and 6). Similarly, several genes that have been identified as candidates for increasing the risk for ASD-related disorders clearly play important roles in fetal brain development. Thus, brain development is altered very early in the development of autism.

And, as discussed in chapter 5, although the overt, psychotic symptoms in schizophrenia are not manifest until early adulthood, it is highly likely that the disorder begins in the early stages of brain development. Structural MRI reveals neuropathology prior to psychosis, and many behavioral abnormalities can be detected in early childhood among subjects who will go on to be diagnosed with schizophrenia. Moreover, epidemiologic studies of environmental risk factors, such as maternal infection, indicate that the window of vulnerability is late in the first half of pregnancy. Similarly, several of the candidate genes for schizophrenia are important for fetal brain development. For instance, Alcino Silva and colleagues at the University of California at Los Angeles made a mouse model in which the function of the gene *DISC1* (*disrupted in schizophrenia 1*; see chapter 6) can be blocked at any stage in the life of the animal. They showed that when the gene is blocked during early development there are much more serious consequences for later abnormal behavior than when the gene is blocked in the adult. As in autism, then, brain circuits are very likely disrupted early in brain development in schizophrenia.

Despite all these observations pointing to the critical importance of embryonic development, studies in animal models of a variety of neurodevelopmental disorders indicate that it is indeed possible to intervene successfully in the adult to restore at least some of the functions lost during development. Moreover, several of these biologically based therapies have proceeded to clinical trials testing their efficacy in adults or children with some of the disorders.

DISC1

As discussed in chapter 6, disruption of the gene for DISC1 can cause major depressive disorder, bipolar disorder, or schizophrenia. Moreover, mouse models of DISC1 disruption can display behavioral abnormalities resembling those in either schizophrenia or depression, depending on the particular mutation in the gene that is introduced into the mice. These mutant mice also display abnormalities in embryonic brain development. Nonetheless, experiments on *adult* mice show that the medications used for human schizophrenia and major depressive disorder can be effective in reversing the behavioral deficits typical for those disorders in the corresponding DISC1 mutants. That is, despite the presumed miswiring of brain circuits that occurred during early development, behavior can be corrected in the adult. These results also indicate that the mouse model can be used in efforts to develop novel, more effective medications. Recall from chapter 6 that antipsychotic medications are effective also in treating and even preventing symptoms when given to adult or adolescent offspring in the maternal immune activation model.

Fragile X

Fragile X syndrome (FXS) is caused by mutations in the FMR1 gene, which is located on the X chromosome. The disease is characterized by a number of symptoms in common with autism, as well as by learning and cognitive deficits, attention deficit hyperactivity disorder, and epilepsy. This devastating disorder is being studied in mouse and *Drosophila* (fruit fly) animal models, where positive preclinical results with several types of novel treatments have led to some promising results in human clinical trials. FXS appears to be one of several ASD-related disorders that exhibit an imbalance between excitation and inhibition in brain circuitry. Too much inhibition means that we sometimes cannot move when we want to (as in Parkinson's disease), while too much excitation means that we move when we do not want to (as in Huntington's disease). In the case of FXS, experiments in the mouse model indicate that there is too much excitation, which leads to deficits in cognitive function. In the *Drosophila* model, lowering the level of excitation with a drug that inhibits binding of a common excitatory neurotransmitter to its receptor rectifies memory deficits and defective courtship behavior as well as structural abnormalities in the central nervous system. Whereas treatment during development corrects all of these deficits, treatment only in adulthood partially ameliorates the courtship and memory deficits without changing the observed structural abnormalities in the brain.

The ability to correct some of the behavior by treatment in the adult is encouraging, even if the structural abnormalities are not reversed. It suggests that rectifying the excitatory/inhibitory imbalance is enough, even with a defective circuit. In fact, these results may mean that excitatory/inhibitory imbalance is the critical feature of the defective circuit. Moreover, experiments in the mouse model also reveal that a similar pharmacological treatment in adulthood can reverse some of the symptoms, such as anxiety in the open-field test and susceptibility to seizures. These results were sufficient to prompt small clinical trials using medications that have effects similar to those tested in the mice. Even though these medications are used to change the excitatory/inhibitory balance, which seems like an inherently risky approach to take, there is evidence that they are safe at the appropriate doses. The trials yielded positive results, improving a variety of deficits in the patients. However, since these were not double-blind trials, the patients knew they were getting the medication, which makes it impossible to rule out a placebo effect. Nonetheless, it is encouraging that positive results were obtained, and more definitive trials are under way. In fact, results from one double-blind trial are positive for a genetically defined subset of patients. Clinical trials are also under way to test two other types of medications, unrelated to the excitatory/inhibitory balance, but which worked well in animal models of FXS.

Rett Syndrome
Rett syndrome (RTT; also discussed in chapter 4) is another genetic disorder that displays a wide variety of symptoms, some of which resemble those found in autism. The patients, who are almost entirely females, appear to develop normally for 6 to 18 months, but this is followed by ASD symptoms, severe mental retardation, seizures, and symptoms characteristic of RTT such as stereotyped hand movements, abnormal breathing, motor deficits, and scoliosis. The mutation causing the disease is in the gene *MeCp2* (which codes for the protein MECP2). In the female mouse model of MeCp2 disruption, which resembles the human syndrome more closely than the male mouse model does, the mice appear to develop normally until about 16 weeks of age (a mouse typically is mature by 4 weeks and dies at 2 to 3 years). The symptoms include motor deficits (such as abnormal walking patterns), breathing abnormalities, tremor, learning deficits, increased anxiety, and stereotyped limb movements. Although this time course indicates a regression, it does not resemble the time course of the regressive form of autism. The female mice are fully adult when symptoms appear, whereas regression in autism typically begins at around 3 years of age. There are also a number of assays for ASD-like behaviors as well as

neuropathology (described in chapter 6) that remain to be conducted in these mice.

In one version of the RTT mouse model, it is possible to disrupt MeCp2 function and then turn the gene back on at any desired time. This feature enabled Adrian Bird and colleagues at the University of Glasgow in Scotland to test the effect of restoring MeCp2 production in adulthood. Remarkably, turning MeCp2 function back on in adult female mutant mice that already express the series of symptoms just described results in restoration of many aspects of behavior, albeit not quite to that of normal mice (figure 9.1). These findings are very important because they offer proof of principle that RTT can be nearly fully reversed (as far as the tested symptoms go, at least) after symptom onset.

These remarkable results raise the question of whether gene therapy is a feasible approach in this disorder. That is, since the MeCp2 gene is mutated in RTT, would giving the patient a normal MeCp2 gene restore normal behavior? In this mouse experiment, a normal MeCp2 gene was "turned back on" genetically, restoring its function. An experiment in actual gene therapy would involve, for example, injecting a virus that

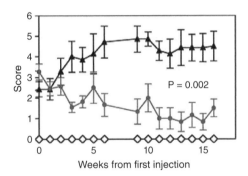

Figure 9.1
In a mouse model, disabling the gene that is affected in human Rett syndrome produces a series of behavioral symptoms that can be quantified by severity as shown on the vertical axis. The scores of the mutant mice are shown by the black triangles. The scores of normal, nonmutant mice are shown by the open diamonds. When the disabled gene is turned back on in adult mutant mice, the symptoms are significantly ameliorated (gray dots). The horizontal axis shows the number of weeks following restoration of gene function. $P = 0.002$ indicates that the differences in scores between the mutant and the restored mutant are highly significant. (From Guy et al., 2007)

codes for the normal MeCp2 gene into the brain of a mouse that lacks the functional gene. One difficulty with such an approach is that the virus would have to deliver the gene to the appropriate set of neurons that control the many behaviors of interest. An even more challenging difficulty for RTT, in particular, is that a precise level of MeCp2 must be achieved; both animal and human studies have shown that too little as well as too much of this protein can cause symptoms (albeit different symptoms). Restoration of the correct, normal levels of MeCp2 in the genetic experiment of Bird and colleagues was possible because the normal gene was reactivated and allowed to function as it normally would. In a gene therapy setting, however, neurons would be infected by a virus carrying the gene, and some neurons might be infected by multiple viruses while others might not be infected at all. Only time will tell if these problems can be solved in such experiments using the mouse model.

In light of this work and its challenges, a number of groups are testing other potential therapeutic approaches in RTT mice (see, for example, the Web site of the Rett Syndrome Research Trust). One interesting idea is to restore growth factors that are abnormally low in RTT. Since low brain weight is common in RTT, and neurons in these brains are smaller and extend fewer processes than normal, it is possible that growth factors known to play a role in embryonic brain development are part of the problem in RTT. In fact, measurements of one such protein, insulin-like growth factor-1 (IGF-1), in the cerebral spinal fluid indicate that there is a deficit in children with autism compared to typically developing children. Moreover, the size of the head (and presumably the brain) correlates with the level of IGF-1 in the autism subjects. Therefore, it was of interest to determine the effects of raising IGF-1 levels in the RTT model mice in which the MeCp2 gene is knocked out. When Mriganka Sur and colleagues at the Massachusetts Institute of Technology administered an IGF-1 peptide daily to the mutant mice, starting at 2 weeks of age (equivalent to childhood in humans), they found that it improved locomotor function, partially alleviated breathing and heart rate problems, and even increased life span by 50%. There were also several signs of increased neuronal maturation in the brain. Although the treated mice still developed all of the symptoms seen in the untreated mutant mice, and they still died prematurely, all of these measures were considerably improved by IGF-1 administration. Similar findings have been achieved by increasing the level of another growth factor, brain-derived neurotrophic factor (BDNF). These several results support the strategy of promoting the growth and maturity of the brain as a therapy for RTT, and such a strategy could also be relevant for autism. Recall, however, that autism is characterized by early brain *overgrowth*, the opposite of what happens in RTT. A clinical trial testing IGF-1 in RTT patients was begun in 2009.

Still another intriguing approach for RTT is termed *environmental enrichment* (EE). Certainly, modifying the environment of children with RTT or autism by, for example, reducing stress, can have positive effects on outcome. What is meant by EE in experiments with rodents is to rear them in groups, in relatively large enclosures, with a wide variety of objects to explore (e.g., tunnels, toys, stairs; see box 9.1), as well as running wheels on which to exercise. (Mice will voluntarily run several miles per night with access to such wheels.) This environment is in contrast to the usual rodent housing in which they have free access to food and water but little opportunity for sensory stimulation. In the case of RTT, applying EE to the MeCp2 mutant mice revealed that several aspects of the disease phenotype can be improved. Moreover, levels of brain BDNF and IGF-1 are increased by EE. While EE does not restore normal behavior or lifespan to the RTT mice, it does induce some significant positive effects.

Box 9.1
The Many Positive Effects of an Enriched Environment

A pioneer in the study of learning and neuropsychology, the Canadian Donald Hebb was the first to publish reports on the effects of EE. He brought home some laboratory rats as pets for his children, allowing them free exploration of his home. When he returned them to the lab he found that they showed better problem-solving ability than the lab rats that had been maintained in standard cage housing. The idea behind EE is to rear animals such as rodents and monkeys in a more naturalistic setting. In the wild, it seems likely that activity in rodents is driven primarily by the necessity to find food and mates and to protect territory. The EE setting in the laboratory also offers an additional opportunity for play and the exercise of innate curiosity (figure 9.2).

The effects of EE have been studied in a variety of mouse models of neurological diseases such as Alzheimer's, Parkinson's, and Huntington's diseases, with many positive impacts on symptoms—improvements in learning and

Box 9.1
(continued)

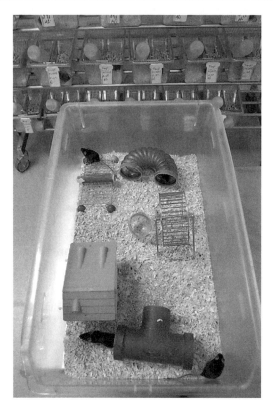

Figure 9.2
An example of an enriched environment (front) versus standard housing (rear) for mice. (From Laviola et al., *Neurobiology of Disease* 31:159–168, 2008)

memory, locomotor activity, and coordination. Amelioration of depressive- and schizophrenia-like behaviors has also been seen. For instance, in experimental epilepsy, when young rats are placed for a time in an enriched environment immediately after a seizure, their immobility in the forced swim test is considerably lessened. Only 10 days in an EE attenuates the depressive-like behavioral symptom caused by seizure. The EE treatment also restores normal levels of the serotonin receptor type 5B, which is depressed by seizure. These findings are clinically relevant because depression is the most frequent psychiatric feature associated with epilepsy. The suicide rate is 20 times higher in people with epilepsy compared with the general population. Conversely,

Box 9.1

(continued)

major depressive disorder increases the risk for unprovoked seizures and the development of epilepsy.

Even in normal, nondiseased mice, EE increases brain weight and the size of neurons, the extension of their processes, and the number of synaptic connections they make with other neurons. These effects of EE are most significant when it is administered during brain development, but there are also positive effects of EE in adult rodents. For instance, EE can increase the production of new neurons the adult brain. Moreover, EE can reduce the cognitive decline associated with aging. This is the effect expressed by the dictum "use it or lose it" in the fields of both developmental neurobiology and brain aging.

Most rodent studies include a running wheel in the EE condition and do not separate the potential positive effects of exercise from those of the stimulating sensory environment. In one experiment aimed at this question, Fred Gage and his colleagues at the Salk Institute in La Jolla, California showed that exercise on the running wheel could account for the EE-induced increase in the production of new neurons in the adult mouse brain. Wheel-running also decreases signs of neuropathology in mouse models of Alzheimer's disease, and improves motor deficits in models of Huntington's disease. Wheel-running prevents and can even reverse the depressive- and anxiety-like behaviors that are induced by stress, effects that are correlated with changes in the level of the serotonin transporter and serotonin receptors. Thus, it seems that exercise alone may be responsible for some of the effects of EE. A caveat for this interpretation is that we do not know whether the rodent also increases its mental activity while running.

Exercise in young rodents also increases the size of certain brain areas, and this effect likely applies to children as well. In new studies from the research group led by Charles Hillman at the University of Illinois it was shown that 9- and 10-year-old children with higher levels of physical fitness score better on cognitive tests and also have larger areas of the brain associated with executive function and memory. The experimenters ruled out other differences among the less and more fit groups of children as being responsible for the brain differences. In a more direct test of the effects of exercise, it was found that just 20 minutes of aerobic activity before a cognitive test elevated scores, even among unfit or overweight children. These results are consistent with the findings on 18-year-old military conscripts in Sweden. Georg Kuhn of the University of Gothenburg reported that better fitness correlated with higher IQ scores, even between identical twins.

There is also ample evidence for positive effects of exercise in the aged population. Physical activity improves cognitive scores and reduces brain

Box 9.1
(continued)

atrophy and the incidence of dementia. There is even some evidence for increased volume in some brain areas.

While exercise appears to mediate some of the effects of EE, sensory stimulation is also likely to play a role. For instance, olfactory enrichment can be achieved in the adult mouse by blowing a variety of fragrances through the cage on a consistent basis. This type of sensory stimulation is sufficient to increase the production of new neurons in the olfactory system. Similarly, it is possible to specifically stimulate the auditory system by playing a variety of sounds. This is sufficient to enhance the function of the auditory system by, for instance, increasing its ability to discriminate between different sounds. In humans, functional MRI has shown that in violin players a greater than normal part of the brain is devoted to the sensory system serving the fingers. A similar phenomenon is observed in monkeys that are rewarded for keeping a finger touching a point on a rotating wheel.

The above experiments were done with adult animals. Recall from chapter 4 that early postnatal tactile stimulation can compensate for inadequate maternal care in the development of, for instance, the ability to respond well to stress. In a recent, rather surprising experiment it was found that daily administration of artificial tactile stimulation to rat pups promotes the development of the visual system. A combination of gently massaging and stroking is effective in accelerating the maturation of the visual cortex in the brain. This is a cross-modal phenomenon, since tactile stimulation activates the somatosensory part of the brain, and the effect being measured is in the visual system. Surprisingly, the tactile stimulation increases the level of IGF-1 in the visual cortex. Moreover, as in the case of the EE experiments on visual system development, blocking IGF-1 action prevents the positive effects of massage.

Similar effects can be seen in humans as well (figure 9.3). For instance, Lamberto Maffei and colleagues at the Institute of Neuroscience in Pisa, Italy, found that massage therapy accelerates brain development in healthy preterm infants, as evaluated by electroencephalography measurements and tests of visual function. Moreover, blood levels of IGF-1 are elevated by massage therapy!

It does seem likely that the results with EE also have implications for human subjects; however, the typical human environment is not as impoverished as the standard housing in cages experienced by laboratory rodents. That is, the difference between EE and standard cage housing may be more extreme than that provided by our manipulation of typical human environments. On the other hand, studies have shown that children of lower

Box 9.1
(continued)

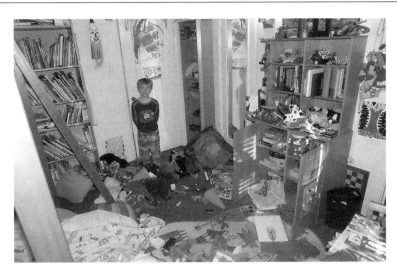

Figure 9.3
An example of an enriched environment for a human. (From P. H. Patterson)

economic status experience far less intellectual stimulation than typical middle-class children. There is also evidence that lack of stimulation during early childhood (deprivation such as was found in Romanian orphanages some years ago) delays and impairs cognitive development. Moreover, people who maintain higher levels of mental and physical activity (as estimated by educational level, engagement in active hobbies, or the type of employment) display greater resistance to the effects of aging and dementia. In addition, a life history of high mental activity correlates with a reduction in age-related atrophy of the hippocampus, a part of the brain involved in learning and memory. Even cancer progresses more slowly in mice housed under EE conditions, and fewer tumors form as well.

And the chasm between regular lab habitat and EE conditions may not be as wide as it first appears, if we remember that although laboratory mice normally live under conditions of sensory deprivation, they are free of the stress of a constant need to find food and water, the necessity to defend their territory, and the danger of predators. In addition, laboratory rodents have access to excellent health care, unlike their counterparts in the wild—or many humans, for that matter.

Environmental enrichment has also been tested using a different mouse model of autistic features, one that is produced by maternal valproic acid (VPA) administration. VPA is used as a medication for treating depression and epilepsy, and is known to cause birth defects. When a woman is taking VPA for such a condition and continues with the medication not realizing she is pregnant, the risk for autism and other problems in her offspring is greatly increased. Thus, VPA is an environmental risk factor that, like maternal infection, poses a threat for autism during early embryonic development. To model this risk in animals, pregnant rats are given VPA, and the offspring exhibit a series of behavioral abnormalities characteristic of autism (such as those described in chapter 6). In one interesting experiment, such offspring were raised under EE conditions for just one week (postnatal days 7 to 14), and then given a series of behavioral tests as adults. Compared to VPA offspring raised under standard housing conditions, the VPA-EE offspring display striking improvements in anxiety, stereotyped behaviors, social interaction, and prepulse inhibition (these tests are described in chapter 6). It is striking that in this experiment, done by Tomasz Schneider and colleagues at the Polish Academy of Sciences in Krakow, the therapeutic effects of EE administered during the rat equivalent of childhood persists through adulthood.

Neurofibromatosis

Mutations in the gene that causes neurofibromatosis type 1 (NF1; the gene *NF1* codes for the protein neurofibromin) cause learning and memory deficits as well as problems with selective attention. These cognitive disabilities can be reproduced in mice that have one copy of the *NF1* gene knocked out. Since neurofibromin is critical for neurodevelopment, it is thought that neurofibromatosis type 1 is a developmental disorder. Nonetheless, recent work from the group of Alcino Silva at the University of California at Los Angeles shows that these cognitive functions can be restored by therapeutic intervention in *adult NF1*-mutant mice. Interestingly, statin medications, which are routinely prescribed for high cholesterol in humans, were used to attenuate learning and memory as well as attention deficits in the NF1 mouse mutants. How are the statins working in this case? There is evidence that they alter the lipid attachment to an important protein in a way that compensates for the change caused by the neurofibromin deficit. That is, the NF1-mutant mouse has an alteration in the lipid attachment to a key protein, and this lipid is restored by statin treatment.

Given the striking results in the mouse model, a pilot clinical trial was carried out in a double-blind manner, in which the statin medication simvastatin or a placebo was given to children with the NF1 disorder for 12 weeks. Although this is a brief treatment duration for a clinical trial, in the mouse model only a short time course of statin administration was needed to reverse symptoms. Although performance on several cognitive tests in the human trial were not improved by the statin, a positive effect was found on the score of one task. With this glimmer of hope, and because the medication has been proven safe for the vast majority of adults, larger trials are being undertaken. This research too could eventually be relevant for autism, since there are reports that NF1 patients can display symptoms of ASD.

It has been surprising and very encouraging to find that it is possible to reverse or prevent symptom onset in the RTT, NF1, and FXS mouse models. However, it should be noted that intervening in the adult has its drawbacks. Most important, years of training during the key period of early childhood have already been lost. Nonetheless, even partial success in adults would be a major step forward, and success in adults could point the way forward to early treatment following initial diagnosis in child-hood. This line of research is also being pursued for other neurodevelop-mental disorders, and it has been possible to prevent symptom onset in mouse models of Down syndrome, tuberous sclerosis complex, and Rubinstein-Taybi syndrome (see the review by Ehninger et al., 2008).

There is another scenario on the horizon: at least 32 different mutations have been found that can make normal mice *smarter* in cognitive tests. Thus, it is possible to explore mechanisms that could someday be used to enhance brain function even in people without learning disorders. Could this lead to a situation similar to that seen in the sports world, where performance-enhancing drugs such as steroids are being banned? Will people in lower economic brackets be at even greater disadvantage if they lack access to medications that enhance mental abilities?

In summary, a substantial fraction of schizophrenia (and possibly autism) incidence could be prevented by the use of appropriate precautions against maternal infection during pregnancy. Public health officials should undertake a campaign to educate the public about this risk factor. The second important conclusion of this chapter is that recent studies of animal models of a variety of neurodevelopmental disorders, including several with relevance to autism and schizophrenia, have shown that it is possible to reverse symptoms—at least partially—using biological interventions. These therapeutic strategies are based on a growing understanding of the neurobiology of the disorders as well as on knowledge about normal embryonic development. If scientists' grasp of the molecular mechanisms underlying these disorders continues to rapidly improve, we can expect to see more effective therapeutics coming from entirely new directions.

Perspectives

A conclusion is the place where you get tired of thinking.
—Arthur Bloch

In this book we have explored a subset of the many and varied ways in which the immune and nervous systems interact. Signals between the two systems can result in nearly immediate effects, as when peripheral infection excites the vagus nerve, which immediately alerts the brain. Brain-immune interactions can also have slower, longer-lasting effects, as when stress induces changes in cortisol receptor levels in the hippocampus, which alters the response to subsequent stress. Some interactions even have permanent consequences, such as the effects of maternal infection on the fetal brain. We have also considered some transgenerational effects—appearing in grandchildren—for instance, involving the inheritance of maternal care behaviors or the effects of maternal malnutrition. Some effects are mediated by epigenetic modifications of the DNA, while others are mediated by molecules that are used in common by neurons and immune cells, such as cytokines and MHC proteins.

The results of this bidirectional communication influence behavior, mood, and cognition, as well as immune function. Examples of behaviors regulated by immune status include sleep, eating, and socialization. The most extreme examples of changes in mood are the symptoms of major depressive disorder, which can be induced by increases in cytokines in the blood. Cognitive functions influenced by immune status include learning and memory and attention. Conversely, immune functions are regulated by the brain during stress. There is also the still mysterious three-way connection between the gastrointestinal tract, the brain, and the immune system, wherein all three influence each other.

The second half of the book deals primarily with the role of the immune system and immune-related molecules in the brain in autism, schizophrenia, and major depressive disorder. Particularly in autism and schizophrenia, there is a great deal of evidence indicating that the brain is in a state of immune activation, and that the peripheral immune system is dysregulated as well. The available evidence suggests that this immune activation could begin in the fetus. That is, a number of environmental risk factors for schizophrenia raise the level of the cytokine IL-6 in the maternal circulation. Animal experiments show that this increase then activates the production of this cytokine in the fetal brain as well as the placenta. We also touched on several examples in which an environmental risk factor can interact synergistically with particular genes.

We have seen evidence that both antibodies and cytokines can mediate the pathological effects of immune activation, and that this can occur both during gestation and in adulthood. We have also discussed the questions that such evidence raises about the effects of vaccination, both in pregnant women and in young children.

Finally, there are several reasons for optimism. Epidemiologic studies are identifying environmental risk factors, many of which can be minimized by way of commonsense precautions. Genetic studies are beginning to identify some mutations that are involved in autism and schizophrenia, as well as common variants of genes that may raise the risk. Study of animal models of these various risk factors is also leading to a far better understanding of the molecular, cellular, and behavioral features of *normal* brain function. Moreover, evidence from animal models is leading to a number of promising clinical trials for treatment of a variety neurodevelopmental disorders. There is hope!

Further Reading

1 Fever and Madness

Almond D (2006) Is the 1918 influenza pandemic over? Long-term effects of *in utero* influenza exposure in the post-1940 U.S. population. *J Political Economy* 114:672–712.

Kolata G (1999) *Flu*. Simon and Schuster, 330 pp.

Morens DM, Taubenberger JK, Fauci AS (2009) The persistent legacy of the 1918 influenza virus. *New Engl J Med* 361:225–9.

Shorter E (1997) *A History of Psychiatry: From the Era of the Asylum to the Age of Prozac*. John Wiley & Sons, pp. 190–239.

Valenstein ES (1986) *Great and Desperate Cures: The Rise and Decline of Psychosurgery and Other Radical Treatments for Mental Illness*. Basic Books, pp. 36–44.

2 Brain-Immune Connections, Stress, and Depression

Belmaker RH, Agam G (2008) Major depressive disorder. *New Engl J Med* 358:55–68.

Boulanger, LM (2009) Immune proteins in brain development and synaptic plasticity. *Neuron* 64:93–109.

Caspi A, Hariri AR, Holmes A, Uher R, Moffitt TE (2010) Genetic sensitivity to the environment: The case of the serotonin transporter gene and its implications for studying complex diseases and traits. *Am J Psychiatry* 167:509–27.

Krebs CJ, Boonstra R, Boutin S, Sinclair ARE (2001) What drives the 10-year cycle of snowshoe hares? *Bioscience* 51:25–35.

Miller G, Chen E, Cole SW (2004) Health psychology: Developing biologically plausible models linking the social world and physical health. *Annu Rev Psychol* 60: 501–24.

Pitychoutis PM, Papadopoulou-Daifoti Z (2010) Of depression and immunity: Does sex matter? *Internl J Neuropharmacol* 13:675–89.

Sloan EK, Captanio JP, Cole SW (2008) Stress-induced remodeling of lymphoid innervation. *Brain Behav Immun* 22:15–21.

3 The Battleground of the Fetal-Maternal Environment

Berger H, de Waard F, Molenaar Y (2000) A case of twin-to-twin transfusion syndrome in 1617. *Lancet* 356:847–8.

Deverman B, Patterson PH (2009) Cytokines and fetal brain development. *Neuron* 64:61–78.

Dulac C (2010) Brain function and chromatin plasticity. *Nature* 465:728–35.

Gartner K (1990) A third component causing random variability beside environment and genotype: A reason for the limited success of a 30 year long effort to standardize laboratory animals? *Lab Animal* 24:71–7.

Gluckman P, Hanson M (2005) *The Fetal Matrix: Evolution, Development and Disease.* Cambridge University Press, 256 pp.

Mor G (2008) Inflammation and pregnancy: The role of toll-like receptors in trophoblast-immune interaction. *Ann NY Acad Sci* 1127:121–8.

Patterson, PH (2007) Maternal effects on schizophrenia risk. *Science* 318:576–7.

Tolkuhn J, Xu X, Shah NM (2010) A custody battle for the mind: Evidence for extensive imprinting in the brain. *Neuron* 67:359–62.

Trowsdale J, Betz AG (2006) Mother's little helpers: Mechanisms of maternal-fetal tolerance. *Nature Immunol* 7:241–6.

Wilkinson LS, Davies W, Isles AR (2007) Genomic imprinting effects on brain development and function. *Nature Rev Neurosci* 8:832–43.

4 Prenatal Origins of Adult Health and Disease

Abel KM, Wicks S, Susser ES, Dlaman C, Pedersen MG, Mortensen PB, Webb RT (2010) Birth weight, schizophrenia, and adult mental disorder. Is risk confined to the smallest babies? *Arch Gen Psychiatry* 67:923–30.

Gliboff S (2006) The case of Paul Kammerer: Evolution and experimentation in the early 20th century. *J History Biol* 39:525–63.

Glucksman PD, Hanson MA, Buklijas T (2010) A conceptual framework for the developmental origins of health and disease. *J Devel Origins Health Dis* 1:6–18.

Heijmans BT, Tobi EW, Lumey LH, Slagboom PE (2009) The epigenome: Archive of the prenatal environment. *Epigenetics* 4:526–31.

Meaney MJ, Szyf M, Seckl JR (2007) Epigenetic mechanisms of perinatal programming of hypothalamic-adrenal-pituitary function and health. *Trends Molec Med* 13:269–77.

Petronis A (2010) Epigenetics as a unifying principle in the aetiology of complex traits and diseases. *Nature* 465:721–7.

Shelton RC, Miller AH (2010) Eating ourselves to death (and despair): The contribution of adiposity and inflammation to depression. *Progr Neurobiol* 91:275–99.

Vargas AO (2009) Did Paul Kammerer discover epigenetic inheritance? A modern look at the controversial midwife toad experiments. *J Exp Zool (Mol Dev Evol)* 312B:667–78.

Zoghbi HY (2003) Postnatal neurodevelopmental disorders: Meeting at the synapse? *Science* 302:826–30.

5   Infections and Behavior

Brown AS, Derkits EJ (2010) Prenatal infection and schizophrenia: A review of epidemiologic and translational studies. *Am J Psychiatry* 167:261–80.

Brown AS, Patterson PH (2011) *The Origins of Schizophrenia*. Columbia University Press, in press.

Webster JP (2007) The effect of *Toxoplasma gondii* on animal behavior: Playing cat and mouse. *Schiz Bull* 33:752–6.

Yolken RH, Torrey EF (2008) Are some cases of psychosis caused by microbial agents? A review of the evidence. *Molec Psychiatry* 13:470–9.

6   Animal Models of Autism, Schizophrenia, and Depression?

Doupe A, Kuhl PK (1999) Birdsong and human speech: Common themes and mechanisms. *Annu Rev Neurosci* 22:567–631.

Hsiao E, Bregere C, Malkova N, Patterson PH (2011) Modeling features of autism in rodents. In *Autism Spectrum Disorders*, ed. Amaral DG, Dawson G, Geschwind DH. Oxford University Press, in press.

Kellendonk C, Simpson EH, Kandel ER (2009) Modeling cognitive endophenotypes of schizophrenia in mice. *Trends Neurosci* 32:347–58.

Patterson PH (2009) Immune involvement in schizophrenia and autism: Etiology, pathology and animal models. *Behav Brain Res* 204:313–21.

Silverman JL, Yang M, Lord C, Crawley JN (2010) Behavioral phenotyping assays for mouse models of autism. *Nature Rev Neurosci* 11:490–502.

Smith SEP, Li J, Garbett K, Mirnics K, Patterson PH (2007) Maternal immune activation alters fetal brain development through interleukin-6. *J Neurosci* 27:10695–702.

7 Immune Involvement in Autism, Schizophrenia, and Depression

Atladótiir HO, Pedersen MG, Thorsen P, Mortensen PB, Deleuran B, Eaton WW, Parner ET (2010) Association of family history of autoimmune diseases and autism spectrum disorders. *Pediatrics* 124:687–94.

Buie T et al. (2010) Evaluation, diagnosis, and treatment of gastrointestinal disorders in individuals with ASDs: A consensus report. *Pediatrics* 125:S1–18.

Careaga M, Van de Water J, Ashwood P (2010) Immune dysfunction in autism: a pathway to treatment. *J Amer Soc Exper NeuroTherapeutics* 7:283–92.

Curran LK, Newschaffer CJ, Lee L–C, Crawford SO, Johnston MV, Zimmerman AW (2007) Behaviors associated with fever in children with autism spectrum disorders. *Pediatrics* 120:e1386–92.

Eaton WW, Byrne M, Ewald H, Mors O, Chen C-Y, Agerbo E, Mortensen PB (2006) Association of schizophrenia and autoimmune diseases: Linkage of Danish National Registers. *Am J Psychiatry* 163:521–8.

Garbett K, Ebert PJ, Mitchell A, Lintas C, Manzi B, Mirnics K, Persico AM (2008) Immune transcriptome alterations in the temporal cortex of subjects with autism. *Neurobiol Dis* 30:303–11.

Janssen DGA, Caniato RN, Verster JC, Baune BT (2010) A psychoneuroimmunological review on cytokines involved in antidepressant treatment response. *Human Psychopharmacol* 25:201–5.

Lee JY, Huerta PT, Zhang J, Kowal C, Bertini E, Bolpe BT, Diamond B (2009) Neurotoxic autoantibodies mediate congenital cortical impairment of offspring in maternal lupus. *Nature Med* 15:91–6.

Martin LA, Ashwood P, Braunschweig D, Cabanlit M, de Water JV, Amaral DG (2008) Stereotypies and hyperactivity in rhesus monkeys exposed to IgG from mothers of children with autism. *Brain Behav Immun* 22:806–16.

Miller AH, Maletic V, Raison CL (2009) Inflammation and its discontents: The role of cytokines in the pathophysiology of depression. *Biol Psychiat* 65:732–41.

Pardo CA, Vargas DL, Zimmerman AW (2005) Immunity, neuroglia and neuroinflammation in autism. *Intl Rev Psychiat* 17:485–95.

Singer HS, Morris CM, Gause CD, Gillin PK, Crawford S, Zimmerman AW (2008) Antibodies against fetal brain in sera of mothers with autistic children. *J Neuroimmunol* 194:163–72.

8 Pre- and Postnatal Vaccination: Risks and Benefits

Gerber JS, Offit PA (2009) Vaccines and autism: A tale of shifting hypotheses. *Vaccines* 48:456–61.

Myers MG, Pineda D (2008) *Do Vaccines Cause That? A Guide for Evaluating Vaccine Safety.* Immunizations for Public Health.

Offit PA (2008) *Autism's False Prophets.* Columbia University Press, 298 pp.

Skowronski DM, De Serres G (2009) Is routine influenza immunization warranted in early pregnancy? *Vaccine* 27:4754–70.

9 Reasons for Optimism

Brown AS, Derkits EJ (2010) Prenatal infection and schizophrenia: A review of epidemiologic and translational studies. *Am J Psychiatry* 167:261–80.

Ehninger D, Li W, Fox K, Stryker MP, Silva AJ (2008) Reversing neurodevelopmental disorders in adults. *Neuron* 60:950–60.

Eyles DW, Feron F, Cui X, Kesby JP, Harms LH, Ko P, McGrath JJ, Burne TH (2009) Developmental vitamin D deficiency causes abnormal brain development. *Psychoneuroendocrinology* 34:S247–57.

Guy J, Gan J, Selfridge J, Cobb S, Bird A (2007) Reversal of neurological defects in a mouse model of Rett syndrome. *Science* 315:1143–7.

McGrath JJ, Eyles DW, Pedersen CB, Anderson C, Ko P, Burne TH, Norgaard-Pedersen B, Hougaard DM, Mortensen PB (2010) Neonatal vitamin D status and risk of schizophrenia. *Arch Gen Psychiatry* 67:889–94.

Nithianantharajah J, Hannan AJ (2009) The neurobiology of brain and cognitive reserve: Mental and physical activity as modulators of brain disorders. *Progr Neurobiol* 89:369–82.

Index

Adaptive immune system, 16–17, 24, 27, 100. *See also* Humoral immune system

Addiction, 46

AIDS, 27, 64

Akil, Huda, xii

Almond, Douglas, 1, 2, 57

Alzheimer's disease, 13, 75, 101, 141, 143

Amaral, David, 105

Amygdala, 23, 114

Angelman syndrome, 40

Angiogenic, 31

Aniston, Jennifer, 79

Antonius, Marcus Aurelius, 43

Armed Forces Institute of Pathology, 1, 2

Arthritis, 10, 11, 25, 106, 107, 114

ASD (autism spectrum disorder), 40, 69, 70, 80, 90, 100, 102, 106–108, 124, 126, 136–138, 147. *See also* Autism

Ashwood, Paul, 107

Asthma, 10, 25, 43, 106, 108, 109

Atladotiir, Hjordis, 70

Autism, 7, 11–13, 17, 23, 34, 36, 38–41, 56, 67, 69–72, 74–76, 78, 80, 82, 83, 84, 89, 90, 92, 94, 95, 97, 99–108, 110, 111, 116, 117, 119–127, 129, 132, 133, 135–138, 140, 141, 146–148, 150. *See also* ASD

Autoimmune, 10, 11, 18, 33, 62, 100, 104–116, 126

Barker hypothesis, 44–46. *See also* Barker, David

Barker, David, 43–46. *See also* Barker hypothesis

Baron-Cohen, Simon, 41

Barres, Ben, 13

Bipolar disorder, 12, 78, 89, 90, 136

Bird, Adrian, 139, 140

Birdsong, 81–83

Blastocyst, 29–31, 38

Bleuler, Eugen, 62, 69

Bloch, Arthur, 149

Blood-brain barrier, 14, 105

Brain-derived neurotrophic factor (BDNF), 141

Brandt, Lawrence, 109

Bridges, Sarah, 117

British Columbia Centre for Disease Control, 118

Brown, Alan, 66–68, 130

Butler, Samuel, 43

Caltech (California Institute of Technology), 108, 109

Cambridge University, 41, 44

Campus Bio-Medico, Rome, 104

Cancer, 28, 43, 44, 103, 113, 130, 145

Cannon, Mary, 72

Carroll, Robert, 7
Caspi, Avshalom, 22, 23
Cats, 63, 68, 131
Celecoxib, 115
Centers for Disease Control, 117, 118
Cerebellum, 80, 81, 92
Cerebral spinal fluid (CSF), 7, 17, 22, 100, 102, 103, 111, 115, 117, 124, 140
Cesarean section, 30, 109
Chase, Stella, 70
Child Health Development Study, 67
Choline supplementation, 133, 134
Clarke, Mary, 72
Clostridium, 109
Clozapine, 96
Coe, Christopher, 96
Cole, Steve, 24
Columbia College of Physicians and Surgeons, 66, 67
Complement cascade, 13, 14
Corticosteroid, 10, 19, 26, 85. See also Cortisol
Corticotrophin releasing factor (CRF), 17, 22
Cortisol, 21, 25, 26, 53–55, 85, 86, 113, 149. See also Corticosteroid
Cotton, Henry A., 7
Courchesne, Eric, 135
Crohn's disease, 10
Cystic fibrosis, 68
Cytokine, 10, 12, 14–19, 25–27, 30, 32, 38, 40, 49, 50, 62, 63, 66, 91, 93–95, 99–104, 107, 111–116, 149, 150
Cytomegalovirus, 61, 70

Dantzer, Robert, 14
Darwin, Charles, 58, 59
De Serres, Gaston, 118
Dendritic cell (DC), 31
Depression (major depressive disorder), 3, 7, 9, 17–19, 22, 23, 25–27, 40, 41, 43, 49, 50, 53, 62, 65, 67, 74, 76,

84–90, 99, 103, 112–116, 126, 135–137, 142, 143, 146, 149, 150
Diabetes, 2, 3, 10, 36, 43, 45, 48
Diamond, Betty, 105
Diet, 44, 45, 47–49, 52, 126, 127, 131–134
DISC1 (disrupted in schizophrenia 1), 65, 89, 90, 136, 137
Dizygotic twins, 34, 36–39
Dolphins, 74
Dopamine, 46, 112
Down syndrome, 147
Drosophila, 137
Duke University, 22
Dulac, Catherine, 40
Dutch Hunger Winter, 47, 52, 67

Eaton, William, 111
Ehninger, D., 147
Einstein, Albert, 129
Eliot, T. S., 61
Emory University School of Medicine, 113
Endometrium, 30, 31
Environmental enrichment (EE), 141–146
Epidemiology, 19, 43–45, 49, 65, 67, 69, 106–108, 119, 123, 124, 130–133, 136
Epigenetic, 39, 40, 50–55, 58, 60, 149
Exercise, 45, 50, 113, 141, 143, 144

Fatemi, Hossein, 91
Feldon, Jerome, 92
Ferguson, M., 9
Fever, 3, 4, 6, 7, 14, 17, 103, 106
Folic acid, 51, 52
FOXP2, 83, 84
Fragile X syndrome (FXS), 13, 137, 138, 147
Freedman, Robert, 133
Functional MRI, 23, 79, 107, 135, 144

Gage, Fred, 143
Gastrointestinal (GI) tract, 80, 107–109,
    149. *See also* Gut
Genomic imprinting, 39, 40
GSK3b, 90
Guillain-Barré syndrome, 10, 122
Gut, 15, 107, 109. *See also*
    Gastrointestinal tract
Guy's Hospital, 44

Hallucination, 3, 64, 69, 76, 78–80
Haloperidol, 63
Harvard University, 11, 40, 45
Hebb, Donald, 141
Herd effect, 127
Herpes virus, 61, 68, 130, 131
HERV (human endogenous retrovirus),
    61, 62
Highland Hospital, 7
Hinsie, Leland, 6
Hippocampus, 25–27, 53–55, 85, 86,
    113, 115, 145, 149
HIV, 25, 27, 34, 61, 64
Holy, Tim, 82
HPA axis. *See* Hypothalamic-pituitary-
    adrenal (HPA) axis
Hsiao, Elaine, 15, 26, 48, 95
Hultin, John, 1
Humoral immune system, 24. *See also*
    Adaptive immune system
Huntington's disease, 75, 137, 141, 143
Hygiene, 108, 110, 126
Hypothalamic-pituitary-adrenal (HPA)
    axis, 18, 25, 26, 85, 86, 112, 113

IGF-1, 39, 40, 140, 141, 144
Immediate early gene (IEG), 79, 80
Imperial College London, 62
Influenza, 1, 3, 14, 27, 64–69, 91, 94,
    96, 114, 118–120, 130, 131
Innate immune system, 24, 27, 31, 49,
    100
Institute of Neuroscience, Pisa, 144

Instituto Neurológico de Colombia,
    Bogotá, 101
Interferon-alpha (Ifna), 113–115
Interferon-beta, 25
Interferon-gamma, 73
Interleukin-1 (IL-1), 10, 113
Interleukin-10 (IL-10), 95
Interleukin-18 (IL-18), 40
Interleukin-6 (IL-6), 10, 14, 17, 26, 27,
    49, 50, 93–95, 101, 102, 108, 111,
    113, 114, 150

Jamison, K. R., 73
Jefferson Medical College, 67
Johns Hopkins University, 67, 69, 99,
    101, 103, 111

Kammerer, Paul, 58–60
Kanner, Leo, 69
Keck School of Medicine at the
    University of Southern California,
    108
KE family, 83
Khoruts, Alexander, 109
Kinship theory, 39
Koch, Robert, 3
Kraepelin, Emil, 62

Lamarck, J-B., 58
Lancet, 121
Larsen, Gary, 81
Levitt, Pat, 108
Lipopolysaccharide (LPS), 91, 106
LSD, 79
Lynx, 20, 21

Maffei, Lamberto, 144
Mahler, Alma, 60
Mahler, Gustav, 60
Major histocompatibility complex
    (MHC), 9–13, 34, 71, 99, 101, 107,
    111, 149
Malaria, 4–6, 62

Malkova, Natalia, 81, 82, 92
Malnutrition, 52, 94, 132, 149
Massachusetts Institute of Technology,
   140
Massage therapy, 144
Maternal care, 53–55, 60, 86, 144,
   149
Maternal immune activation (MIA), 72,
   91–96, 108, 110, 134, 137
Maternal infection, 12, 57, 64, 65,
   67–72, 80, 91, 92, 94–97, 108, 110,
   111, 116, 117, 130, 132, 135, 136,
   146, 147, 149
Mazmanian, Sarkis, 108, 109
McAllister, Kim, 95
McGill University, 53
McGrath, John, 132
Meaney, Michael, 53
Measles, 68, 121, 122, 124, 127
MeCp2, 55, 138–141
Mednick, Sarnoff, 65, 67
Mendel, 58, 59, 129
Merck, 122
MET, 108, 120,
Methylation, 51–55, 57, 60
Meyer, Urs, 92, 94, 95
MHC. See Major histocompatibility
   complex (MHC)
Microbes, 7, 9, 10, 14, 15, 24, 31, 38,
   49, 107–109, 116
Microglia, 15, 16, 40, 101, 102, 107
Midwife toad, 58–60
Miller, Andrew, 113
Mirnics, Karoly, 104, 110
MMR vaccine, 121–124
Molecular mimicry, 10, 104, 106,
   111
Monozygotic, 34–39
Montefiore Medical Center, Albert
   Einstein College, 109
MRI, 23, 27, 64, 68, 79, 96, 114, 135,
   136, 144
Mullis, Kary, 99

Multiple sclerosis (MS), 10, 33, 40, 41,
   50, 61, 100, 109, 115
Mumps, 121, 127

National Advisory Committee on
   Immunization, 118
National Alliance for Research on
   Schizophrenia and Depression
   (NARSAD), 67
National Institutes of Health, 67
Natural killer cell (NK), 31
Negative symptoms, 76
Neophobic, 63, 80
Neuregulin, 65
Neurofibromatosis (NF1), 146
Neuroligin, 65
New Jersey State Hospital, 7
New York State Psychiatric Institute, 67
New York University Medical Center,
   70
Noble, G. Kingsley, 60

Oocyst, 63
Oregon Health & Science University,
   44

Paabo, Svante, 83
Pardo, Carlos, 99–101
Parkinson's disease, 46, 101, 137, 141
Parvalbumin, 76, 92
Pasamanic, Benjamin, 65
Patterson, P. H., 74, 129, 145
Pearce, Karen, 135
Persico, Antonio, 104
Placenta, 29–39, 46, 53, 62, 95, 105,
   150
Polio, 121
Polish Academy of Sciences, Krakow,
   146
Poly(I:C), 91–96, 119
Positive symptoms, 76
Positron emission tomography (PET),
   101

Prader-Willi syndrome, 40
Prepulse inhibition, 78, 80, 90, 92, 146
Psoriasis, 50, 114
PTSD, 27
Purkinje cell, 80, 81, 92
Pyrotherapy, 3, 5, 62

Reid, Ann, 1
Retrovirus, 61
Rett syndrome (RTT), 55, 56, 138–141, 147
Royal College of Surgeons, 72
Royal Free Hospital, 121, 122
Rubella (German measles), 68, 70, 71, 121, 127
Rubeola, 70
Rubinstein-Taybi syndrome, 147

Salk Institute, 143
Schizophrenia, 3, 5–7, 11, 12, 23, 34, 36–38, 40, 41, 43, 45–47, 52, 53, 61–72, 73, 74, 76–80, 84, 86, 89–92, 94–97, 99, 110–112, 116, 117, 119–121, 126, 129–137, 142, 147, 148, 150
Schneider, Tomasz, 146
Schwartz, Michal, 115
Seizure, 79–81, 90, 138, 142, 143
Serotonin receptor, 87–89, 142, 143
Serotonin transporter, 22, 87, 88, 143
Shepard, R.W., 9
Shi, Limin, 92
Silva, Alcino, 72, 136, 146
Skowronski, Danuta, 118
Sleeping sickness, 62
Smith, Stephen, 93, 94
Song, 56, 81–83, 92. See also Birdsong
Spanish flu, 1, 119
Spenser, H., 29
Shatz, Carla, 11, 12
Serotonin, 18, 19, 22, 80, 85, 87–89, 142, 143

Selective serotonin reuptake inhibitor (SSRI), 19, 23, 85, 87, 88
Snowshoe hare, 20, 21
SSRI. See Selective serotonin reuptake inhibitor (SSRI)
Stanford University, 11, 13
Statin, 18, 146, 147
Stress, 9, 17–28, 47, 52–55, 57, 80, 84–88, 91, 92, 94, 112, 113, 115, 133, 141, 143–145, 149
Suicide, 18, 49, 55, 60, 115, 142
Sur, Mriganka, 140
Susser, Ezra, 66, 67
Swine flu, 1, 122
Swiss Federal Institute of Technology Zurich, 92
Sympathetic nerve, 23–25, 27
Syphilis, 3, 4, 6
Systemic lupus erythematosus (SLE), 105, 106
Szyf, Moshe, 53

Taubenberger, Jeffrey, 1
T cells, 33
Tel Aviv University, 91
Templeton, W.L., 5, 6
Testosterone, 37, 41, 42
Tetrault, Nicole, 102
Thalidomide, 70, 135
Thimerosal, 122, 124, 125
Thrifty phenotype, 46, 48
Tolerance, 32, 33
Torrey, E. Fuller, 65
Toxoplasma gondii, 62–64, 68, 130
Transgenerational, 47, 54, 149
Tregs, 33
Trophoblast, 30–32, 34
Tuberous sclerosis (TSC) tuberculosis, 3, 6
Tumor necrosis factor-alpha (TNF), 114
Twain, Mark, 117
Twin, 34–38, 41, 47, 65, 143
Twin transfusion syndrome, 35, 36

Ultrasonic vocalization (USV), 81, 82, 84, 90, 92
Universidad Industrial de Santander in Bucaramanga, Colombia, 101
University of Aarhus, 70
University of Birmingham, 44
University of California at Berkeley, 11
University of California at Davis, 105, 107
University of California at Los Angeles, 24, 72, 136, 146
University of California at San Diego, 135
University of Colorado Denver, 133
University of Glasgow, 139
University of Illinois, 14, 143
University of Minnesota, 91
University of Pittsburgh, 67
University of Queensland, 132
University of Southern California, 65
University of Wisconsin, 96
Urinary tract infection, 62, 71, 72
U.S. Advisory Committee on Immunization Practice, 118

Valproic acid (VPA), 135, 146
Vanderbilt University, 104
Van de Water, Judy, 107
Varicella, 70
Vioxx, 122
Vitamin D, 132, 133
Vagus nerve, 14, 15, 17, 149
Vaccination (vaccine), 7, 15, 26, 33, 70, 108, 114–116, 117–127, 131, 132

Wagner-Juaregg, Julius von, 3–5
Wakefield, Andrew, 121–123, 125
Washington University of St. Louis Medical School, 82
Webster, Joanne, 62

Weiner, Ina, 91, 95
Weitzmann Institute, 91
Wisconsin card sorting test, 46

Zimmerman, Andrew, 100, 103